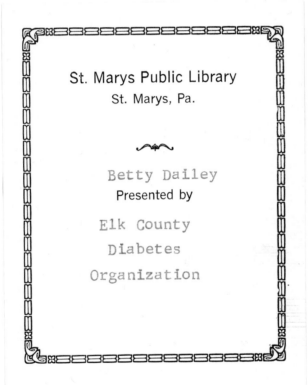

LIVING WITH
A BROKEN STRING

Mary Cooper Greene

Library of Congress Catalog Card Number 87-92172

ISBN 0-9619-9790-7

This book was especially written for insulin-dependent diabetics.

I have written it as a message of hope and encouragement to you.

Do you remember the childhood story of "The Little Engine That Could?" Many times in our diabetic world, we become much like that engine, saying; I think I can, I think I can, but never really knowing for sure.

As you read my personal story, I hope this message rings loud and clear. I know you can, I know you can.

Your friend,

Mary Greene

To my husband, John Sr., who
as critics might say, certainly
took a chance marrying a diabetic!
Thanks for never complaining about
this disease, and for all your help
in controlling it.

A special word of thanks to Gladys and
Wally Uber, Lucille Smith Stanko, and
Bill and Ginny Cooper, for your help
and encouragement while preparing
this manuscript.

Above all, my heartfelt thanks to
Dr. B. Leonard Snider, Dr. Barry D. Stamm,
Dr. John B. Nesbitt, and especially to
Dr. David D. Kirkpatrick Jr., I love you all.

Contents

Preface

Dr. B. Leonard Snider, a dermatologist, who recently removed a basal cell carcinoma (tumor) from my right eyebrow, walked into the room where my husband and I were waiting. Picking up my chart, he remarked about the fact that I was a diabetic. Turning towards me, he asked: "How long have you been a diabetic?"

Half smiling, I replied. "Well, if I live until next November it will be 40 years."

"40 years," he mused. He then began telling us about a friend who had recently been diagnosed with the disease, and was having a problem adjusting, especially to the insulin injections. After some discussion, Dr. Snider stepped back and heartily remarked, "Why don't you write a book?"

My husband and I laughed at his suggestion, and when my examination was finished headed back to our farm.

Spring is a very busy time on any farm, and that year for us was no exception. Our hectic pace continued, yet the remark Dr. Snider made kept running through my mind. There is still much controversy about diabetes, but, oh what I would have given for a book written by a diabetic, someone who actually lived with it, and could have shared with me all the things I questioned.

Diabetes is the third leading cause of death in the United States today, and one out of twenty Americans is now diabetic. Nevertheless, the fears and worries that have been drilled into each and every diagnosed diabetic are often much worse than the disease itself. Just thinking about the villains; blindness, gangrene, kidney failure, and neuropathy is enough to send chills down my spine. However, I think it's time to let people know you can live successfully with this disease.

Looking back at the word disease, I really hate to use it. I often think of disease as something that ravages the body, and diabetes, well controlled, is not that kind of a "problem."

Would I have traded my "problem" for somebody else's if I could have had the choice? Absolutely not! This "problem" has become my friend. We've walked a long way together, and I wouldn't have missed the last 40 years even with diabetes.

As I share my story with you, I cannot separate the physical from the spiritual, they are so interwoven. So I must also share my faith in God. He is my loving Friend and Heavenly Father, and the many promises from God's word intermingled through this book are truly part of me and my life.

At times, we all reach a point where we want to "give up." Yet, as diabetics we really can't afford to give up. There is life beyond diabetes. And we must start each day with a renewed hope and determination to fight this disease . . . whoops, I mean "problem," and win.

"Don't let yesterdays' failures
bankrupt tomorrows' efforts."

CHAPTER 1

She Must Have Been Faking

Fall is my favorite time of year, and the fall of 1947 was no exception. I was ten years old, and beginning the sixth grade at Longfellow Elementary School in Erie, Pennsylvania. We lived on Downing Court, a street filled with neat brick houses, two-and-one-half blocks from the grade school. We did not ride school buses back then, but the walk to school was always fun.

I am the youngest of seven children. My brother Jim is the eldest, then there are my sisters; Gladys, Edith, Ida, Eleanor, and then brother Bill, who is two years older than me. Jim, Gladys, and Edith were married and on their own.

1

We were a close family, and Bill usually made it his business to keep an eye on me. He was really grown up, of course, and now attending the eighth grade at Gridley Junior High School. After school, my friends and I would gather, and while Bill was folding newspapers, listen eagerly to all the fun he was having at Gridley. We were really looking forward to attending junior high school next year.

There were two floors at Longfellow School, and by the middle of September, climbing those stairs exhausted me. It was nothing to bother mother about; she certainly had enough problems. My father, who was a Chief Petty Officer in the United States Navy, had passed away four years before. Cancer, they said. A disease not very common back then.

At a time when most mothers stayed home and raised their children, mine had to go out and work to support her family. She found a job at Weiblen's Pharmacy, a small drug store just a block and a half from our house. Fortunately, it was an easy walk for her, as we did not own a car. Mother seldom complained, and dinner time was always filled with happy experiences from her day. The customers were interesting, and she enjoyed her work.

After graduating from high school, Ida went to work at Loblaws, a large grocery chain. Eleanor and Bill had paper routes to keep them busy after school, so it was always my job to wash and dry the breakfast dishes, and prepare dinner for the family.

Ida planned the menus for me, and purchased the groceries with her paycheck, while mother's pay went towards the other bills, and mortgage on our small brick home.

As I prepared dinner late in September, I

couldn't help but notice how thirsty I was. My, how good the water tasted!

My eleventh birthday came in October, but somehow, I just wasn't feeling good enough to enjoy the party my family had for me. Nothing you could put your finger on; growing pains they called it.

Walking to school soon became a chore for me, and I began complaining of being tired. Everyone had a lot to do, and my older brothers and sisters thought I was just trying to get out of doing my share.

But by late October I could no longer walk to school. I was literally drinking gallons of water and urinating constantly. I laid on the couch during the day, and put the telephone within easy reach, as mother called often to check on me.

My fleeting strength made it difficult for me to do the dishes or fix dinner, and Eleanor had to do it when she returned from her paper route. This didn't make her very happy, as she later told me. "Honey, I thought you were faking."

There were no other symptoms just tiredness, drinking, and urinating. In a short time the thirst got so bad that water no longer satisfied, and a horrible phlegm developed in my throat.

My brother and sisters were happily planning a Halloween party that year. They had a tub set up in the basement to bob for apples with their friends. Of course, they were thinking, a party will surely bring Mary around, but that was one party I could not get excited about. By this time I was almost too weak to make it upstairs to the bathroom.

Mother had talked with Mr. Weiblen, the pharmacist, many times about my condition, but with no other symptoms, he did not think it was anything very serious. Insulin had only been discovered in the 1920's and we very seldom heard of anyone having diabetes, except . . . . my grandmother, my father's mother. I was named after her, and she lived in Philadelphia many miles away.

Thursday evening came, and I could hear the laughter of the young people down in the basement. Oh, what fun they were having! But I distinctly remember that I just didn't care. I was so tired, all I wanted to do was sleep.

The following Sunday I developed a stomachache. By this time I had lost a noticeable amount of weight, and now Eleanor, Ida, and Bill took turns helping me upstairs to the bathroom.

On Monday morning mother made an appointment for me with our family doctor. She had to work until nine o'clock that evening, and since Eleanor was now working at the drug store each Monday night, Ida was responsible for getting me to the doctor's office.

My appointment with Dr. Joseph Walsh was at eight o'clock. Ida and I started out for his office, which was only a block away, but what a struggle she had trying to get me there. I was so weak I could barely walk. She tried carrying me, but her limited strength and size made the task difficult. Fortunately, the man who delivered our dry cleaning each Monday evening saw her predicament, and came to her rescue. However, when we walked in the doctor's office, every seat in the waiting room was taken. A man got up so I could have his chair. "Oh, thank you," I said. How grateful I was.

Dr. Walsh did not have a secretary or a nurse working for him. But soon the door opened, and the doctor stepped out calling a woman's name. The man who had given me his chair went in with the woman. Ida sat down beside me, and held my head on her lap. The next time the door opened, Dr. Walsh said, "Mary, you'd better come in."

Everyone in our neighborhood knew Dr. Walsh, and likewise, he knew most of us. We were neighbors. Ida helped me into his office, where Dr. Walsh lifted me onto his cold table. In the course of his examination the doctor began poking my stomach. "Ouch," it really hurt!

The next thing I knew Dr. Walsh was on the telephone talking to mother at the drug store. I could hear him saying: "Mary must be admitted to the hospital tonight, she has appendicitis!"

Mother immediately called Jim to meet us at the doctor's office. Seemed like only seconds passed, and she was standing beside me. She sent Ida to the drug store to fill in for her, then, mother, Jim, and I were on the road headed for Saint Vincent's Hospital.

Of course, by this time my family was genuinely frightened, but a wonderful promise from God's word, found in Isaiah says:

> Fear thou not, for I am with thee;
> be not dismayed, for I am thy
> God; I will strengthen thee, yea I
> will help thee; yea I will uphold
> thee with the right hand of my
> righteousness.
> Isaiah 41:10.

CHAPTER 2

The Diagnosis

Dr. Walsh arranged my immediate admittance upon arriving at the hospital. Soon, nurses were helping me out of my clothes, and into a hospital gown that hung pitifully on me.

The next thing I knew a man in a clean white jacket was bending over me tying a tight band around my upper right arm. "Mary, make a tight fist for me," he instructed. Obediently, I squeezed my fingers hard. He poked my arm vein with his finger, and drew out the longest needle I'd ever seen in my life!

"Ouch!"

Soon blood was oozing into the tube. As the blood flowed, he released the tight band and drew the needle out.

"Whew, I hope I never have to go through that again," I mused. Little did I realize that was only the beginning of a long series of "ouches."

A nurse then pulled the curtain around my bed saying, "Mary, can you give me a urine specimen?" That I could certainly do.

Within minutes, a surgeon I never became acquainted with examined my stomach. Oh, but I was tired, so I curled up on my side and fell asleep.

"Mary, wake up! I have a shot for you," the nurse exclaimed.

"A what?"

"A shot, dear. Dr. Walsh is with your mother; they will be in shortly." Oh, but I was glad when the shot was over.

Soon, Dr. Walsh and mother walked into my room. It looked like mother had been crying. She stepped over to me and clasped my hand, saying, "Mary, they've found a problem known as diabetes mellitus, and they cannot operate until the diabetes is under control."

"Oh well, mom, don't worry," I whispered. "Everything will be alright."

"But, honey," she continued wistfully, "They can't cure diabetes, at best, they can only try to control it."

"Diabetes," I said to myself, but my thoughts were interrupted by the tired, forlorn expression on mother's face. "Mom, please don't worry, I'll be okay, I'm so tired now I just want to sleep."

With that, I again drifted off into a sound sleep, that is, until I heard a familiar voice saying, "Mary, wake up! I want you to make another fist for me."

"Oh, no, not this again."

Immediately following him a doctor approached, wheeling a pole which had a funny-looking bottle attached to it. A nurse carrying some objects said, "Mary, we want to start an intravenous feeding, will you make a fist for the doctor?"

"Let's use the left arm," the doctor said to the nurse. He was good at it didn't take him long to find a vein. Then, the needle was inserted. A board was placed under my arm, and they wound lots of tape around them both. In just a few minutes that same nurse was back with another shot for me.

"What's that?" I asked.

"Insulin," was her short reply.

All this time mother was sitting close to my bed. She never left the hospital while the entire process of blood and urine testing along with insulin injections continued throughout the night. I'm sure mother must have been very tired, I just wished she wasn't so sad.

As the morning sun streamed through my hospital window, a new nurse walked into my room. She greeted me pleasantly, checked the intravenous, then walked over and felt the back of my neck. I wondered what in the world she did that for?

While a nurse changed my bed sheets, Dr. Walsh walked in. He examined my stomach, and as much poking as he was doing, you'd think it would have hurt like crazy, but odd as it may seem, the stomach pain was gone.

Dr. Walsh straightened up, and with a solemn expression, said; "Mary, I admitted you to the hospital last night for immediate surgery, but the results of the preliminary tests revealed an extremely high blood glucose level. As your mother mentioned last night, this condition is known as diabetes. You're still a very sick little girl, and you will have to remain in the hospital until we get your diabetes under control."

"But what about my appendix?" I questioned.

"Surgery won't be necessary; your appendix is fine," he replied. "You are a very lucky girl. You were only hours away from a diabetic coma, which could have been fatal."

At eleven years of age, my only thought was, "Oh, that's great, I can't wait to tell Eleanor and Bill that I really am sick." However, I just couldn't understand why everyone seemed to be so down-in-the-dumps. I was beginning to feel a little better, and the terrible phlegm that bothered me was not as thick. It no longer was difficult to swallow, and water was starting to taste good again.

As the doctor left, Jim and his wife Florence appeared in the doorway. "We're going to take mom home now, honey, so she can get some rest," Jim said.

"I'll be back tonight." Mom commented, as she kissed my cheek.

"Mom, will you bring my watch with you?"

Mom nodded "yes." I'd received my first watch for Christmas that year. I loved wearing it to school, and now that I was going to be in the hospital awhile I might just as well keep track of the time.

With everyone gone, I thought, "This can't be all that bad." I'd never been in a hospital before, but I was really quite comfortable laying between those clean white sheets. There was always someone checking on me, and they even helped me up on the bedpan. The only thing I couldn't do was get out of bed or move my left arm. Granted, the big board was a nuisance, but it didn't hurt, and the shots weren't all that bad anymore. The only thing I really hated was when they drew blood out of my arm.

I was soon to become familiar with some new terms: Juvenile and insulin-dependent. The term: type I had not been thought of yet. As a diabetic these terms now applied to me. Why was the nurse checking the back of my neck? Of course, you know. However, it was another new term for me: Insulin reaction! I soon learned how to recognize them. At least once each day, and sometimes more, sweat would trickle down my neck and forehead. Then, my fingers pressed down hard on the hospital bell as I rang for orange juice with sugar.

My hospital stay lasted four weeks, quite a long time, but keep in mind, this was 40 years ago. Those of you reading this who are newly diagnosed, were probably only a short time getting in control. For that, you can thank the newly improved insulins, and the excellent knowledge available to your physician today.

My hospital stay was also a complete learning experience, not only for me, but for my family as well. Even the insulin shots I was taught to give myself, though scary at first, turned out fine. I loved practicing on the big, fat orange they gave me. Each morning I alternated legs first my right, then my left, while an experienced nurse supervised the process.

When the nursing supervisor advised that someone else in my family should learn, Ida volunteered. She said everyone else was too frightened. I'm glad it was Ida. I'd sure never let Eleanor or Bill come near me with a needle, especially Bill!

Incidentally, each evening someone from my family was at the hospital to see me. We lived 22 blocks from Saint Vincent's Hospital. However, Gladys and her husband, Wally, took turns with Jim and Florence, picking up mother, Ida, Eleanor, and Bill for nightly visits. They were both building new houses in different suburbs of Erie. It was a great distance for them to drive, especially with all they were doing, but I never once heard anyone complain. In fact, everyone was starting to smile again.

Dear friend, I hope you will always appreciate along with me the adjustment your family made when your diabetes was diagnosed. I never fail to give thanks for the special blessing of a loving family, both my own, and now my chosen family: my husband and son, along with my husband's family. These people would do anything they could to help me, not only with my diabetes, but with any problem I face, and I think this is true in most families.

Just a word to parents of diabetic children: Even after 40 years with this "problem," my heart is still deeply touched whenever I hear of a child diabetic. However, the process of diabetes from discovery to control, is much harder on you, the parent, then it is on your child. How do I know? Remember; I've been there.

As mothers and fathers of diabetic children, I know sometimes your heart is breaking under the strain, and I am often asked, "At what age is a child responsible?" This, of course, depends a great deal on the child's maturity level. From my own experience, if they are age ten or older, and you are still doing most of the control work, such as blood and urine testing along with insulin dispensing, I beg you to please stop!

But you say, that sounds cruel. No, your main responsibility as parents is to make sure your child is thoroughly educated in diabetic management by their physician, or anyone he or she recommends for this learning process. Be sure to attend the instruction with them, but don't interfere. If your child refuses to cooperate, don't let it frustrate you. Sooner or later your child will realize that in order to feel good they must be in good control.

Some parents feel such pity for their diabetic child that without realizing it, they spoil them, especially, when there are other children in the family without this "problem." Parents also tend to blame themselves after their child is diagnosed diabetic, and this is sad.

I'm distressed when I read of parents coping with diseases like cancer in their children. Many times there is "no hope" for that child, however, that is no longer true for the diabetic child.

Other parents convey stories, finally admitting that their diabetic child likes to make life miserable for the rest of the family. This kind of behavior is uncalled for. Our thoughts may differ, but when I misbehaved, I received what the rest of my brothers and sisters got: a good old-fashioned spanking.

Children are very perceptive. They sense your pity and concern, and your acceptance of their diabetes is absolutely necessary.

The Erie County Diabetes Association, of which I am a member, consistently offers a yearly "get together" for parents and diabetic children. One of the certified psychologists conducting this meeting in Erie is Mrs. Wanda Salvia, a personal friend of mine. Wanda has also been a diabetic for quite some time.

I cannot stress enough the importance of meetings like this, because some parents tend to help their diabetic child too much, some too little . . . few just enough.

Wherever you live, I heartily recommend your local Diabetes Association. Take advantage of the interesting programs offered by your local group. You will find wonderful fellowship with others like yourself, and even if it's impossible for you to attend all the meetings, the monthly newsletter offers much information and good recipes shared by other diabetics.

As this chapter ends, I want to share with you one of the wonderful tools I've found personally for healing and control. It is found in the book of Proverbs:

> A joyful heart is good medicine.
> But a broken spirit dries up the
> bones.
>> Proverbs 17:22.

Now that doesn't say discontinue your medication, and eating pattern. Please don't get carried away; but work on a joyful heart. It will do wonders for you, and I might add, it will probably be much appreciated by your doctor the next time you have your checkup.

Everyone was talking, laughing, and wishing me well for today I was going home. Sitting in the wheel chair with my arms loaded with books and games, the head nurse bent down and kissed my cheek. It was then I saw tears in her eyes. I'm quite sure she was wondering if there was any future for this little diabetic girl she had cared for? How would she handle life? Would she live to enjoy teenage years? Adulthood?

If we could each have one wish granted to us in this life, mine would be, that if she is still living, she will read this book, and remember me.

CHAPTER 3

True Friends

Ida took a six week leave of absence from Loblaws so she could watch and supervise me at home. I was not permitted to return to school until classes resumed after Christmas vacation. She also helped me get caught up with the school work I missed.

In mid-January mother accompanied me on my first visit back to Dr. Walsh. While we waited, my thoughts returned to the night my head lay on my sister's lap waiting for him. But today I sat straight and tall in my chair, and how was I feeling? Simply wonderful! Thanks to Dr. F. G. Banting, and C. H. Best, the two Canadian Medical Scientists who discovered insulin. Remember, when those surges of self-pity come, and you really get down in the dumps, that you and I would not be alive today without that discovery.

Dr. Walsh greeted us warmly, and motioned for us to sit down. He faced mother and said, "Mrs. Cooper, I want you to take Mary to this doctor." He scribbled a name and address on a prescription blank, and handed it to mother. He continued, "We discovered Mary's diabetes quite by accident from the pre-surgical tests, and I must admit that when it came to setting up her food and insulin requirements I needed help. I am not a diabetic specialist." He pointed to the prescription blank saying, "Dr. George Stoney is the best in the city of Erie, and I want you to take Mary to him. I'll make the appointment for you."

Now I was sad; Dr. Walsh and I had become quite good friends during his daily hospital visits, and I would really miss him.

In 1947 there were two large hospitals in Erie: Saint Vincents, and Hamot. The doctors did not usually transfer back and forth. This was not a doctor he knew from his own hospital, but one he sought out because of his fine reputation.

As I was growing up, I often thought about Dr. Walsh and what he did that day. It was hard for me to understand at first, but I later realized it was truly a gallant act. Dr. Walsh was indeed my friend.

Dr. Stoney's office was on East 6th Street, which meant we had to take the bus. Mother, of course, was with me for this first appointment. When we walked into the waiting room, why, there was room to sit down, and when the office door opened, a nurse called my name. There wasn't any waiting here. We marched in behind the nurse, and a short, rather large man extended his hand to mother saying, "I'm Dr. Stoney."

As he sat there questioning mother about me, I was sizing him up. "He was really old," I thought, and he didn't smile very much. I'd almost call him a bit cranky. But then a smile crossed his face, and when he smiled he had a wee twinkle in his eyes. "I'd say if he would smile more often he'd make a great Santa Claus."

However, my observations soon stopped as he began asking me questions. Then turning towards mother he said, "The first thing I want you to do is take Mary to a Diabetic School. It begins February 10, at Hamot Hospital. It is from seven o'clock until nine o'clock each evening, and it runs for two weeks. My nurse will enroll you. I want you to make an appointment with me when the course is completed. Bring a urine specimen with you." And he handed mother a prescription blank. "Have Mary get a fasting blood sugar done at Hamot Hospital the morning before her appointment." "Oh no," I groaned, "I thought I was finished with that stuff!"

The Diabetic School was excellent, and for years after, mother sang its praises. However, it was at this school I met my first irritator. You and I are not always going to like everyone we meet on our diabetic walk, and I will refer to her as Miss X.

She was rather young, and I'm not at all sure what her title was, but if you're interested in an 11 year old's opinion, I think she missed her calling with diabetics. I was the only child diabetic in the class, and one evening she cornered mother. I, of course, was standing beside her. Then, she proceeded to inform us that diabetic children rarely lived more than 20 years with this disease, and if they did, the complications associated with it would make life most miserable.

Can you imagine how mother must have felt. I didn't know anything about the long range outlook of this "problem." All I knew was that I felt good since my release from the hospital.

Incidentally, when Miss X spoke, the only word she really knew in our diabetic vocabulary was diet! You could actually see people squirming in their seats while she talked. I often wonder how her presentation affected her career at Hamot Hospital. The dietician was tactful, and excellent in her knowledge of diabetic food planning.

I'm sure I will be criticized for saying this, but the word diet, when used in connection with insulin-dependent diabetics today, is impractical. I am also quite sure that one word alone loses most diabetics before they ever get started on their walk because the fear connected with it is awesome!

The word diet is fine for people needing to shed extra weight. However, for insulin-dependent diabetics, words like food plan and eating pattern are far more effective.

Why, then, is the word "diet" used so extensively by diabetic educators? Before the discovery of insulin, the only possible way they could keep a diabetic alive for any length of time was by a very strict diet. In fact, most diabetics died of starvation.

When I was released from Saint Vincent's Hospital, the diet that accompanied me was very strict. We weighed and measured everything, and I know if it had not been for Dr. Stoney I would never have succeeded.

I also think the word "diet" has been the worst contributor to the ignorance of diabetes by onlookers. Let me explain: Once when I was young, I could have gotten into infinite trouble listening to a well-meaning, but ignorant person. I so clearly remember my young playmate's mother saying, "You're supposed to be on a strict diet," as I struggled to unwrap a small peppermint pattie to keep myself from an on-coming insulin reaction.

"Just look at you," she exclaimed. And I sure was a sight. I'd failed to catch that one in time. Did you ever look at yourself in an insulin reaction? Well, I had sweat dripping down my neck and forehead, and when relief came, I shook from the freezing cold that invaded my body. I ran for home quite terrified by her remark. If it had not been for the loving, caring family behind me, such circumstances could have really played havoc with my control.

I can still hear mother saying, "Don't ever pay attention to what others say. Dr. Stoney knows exactly what he is doing."

She later called the woman to explain, but I think the explanation fell on deaf ears, as I can't ever remember playing with her daughter again.

Don't forget, I am not a doctor, and any advice shared is simply my own reaction as I continue my diabetic walk. Please don't misunderstand me. Proper eating is very important, but we must stick with a plan with which we can easily live.

Improper eating habits can get us into plenty of trouble. Some diabetics are confused when acetone shows in a urine test. If acetone is not treated it results in a condition known as ketosis. This condition can be very harmful if not treated, and can eventually lead to a diabetic coma.

Fat is usually burned as energy or stored as layers of fat. When diabetics eat incorrectly or don't take the proper amount of insulin to utilize the fat, then fragments, known as ketones or acetone, seep into the blood.

However, if diabetics will check themselves carefully, take the proper amount of insulin, and eat regular meals this problem should not occur.

There is a word which insulin-dependent diabetics need to be very aware of. That word is simply; BALANCE.

Incidentally, it you are a Type I or Type II diabetic, and suffer from obesity, I strongly believe you will do much for yourself and your diabetes if you will shed those extra pounds.

Returning to school was great. My friends were glad to see me, and we talked about everything I'd missed, and a lot more. But one subject we never discussed was, yep, you guessed it, diabetes. That was none of their business; a very common reaction in children.

My education with Dr. Stoney continued and I give him all the credit for being the healthy, well-controlled diabetic I am today. I want to share some of his instruction with you.

Each insulin-dependent diabetic is a separate person. We cannot be grouped together for a control program, our lifestyles are completely different. The most successful diabetic today will know THEM-

SELVES well. You and I have a blood sugar level our bodies feel good at. This is always within the normal range. I can hear Dr. Stoney saying over and over again, "Mary, don't ever let your body get used to a constantly high blood sugar." And with that I have been very fortunate.

Remember in chapter one, when I told you about my long, slow acquaintance with a high blood glucose level: the thirst, constant urination, and fatigue? Well, it is a feeling I cannot stand! It should not take any diabetic long to recognize the symptoms, as they always remain the same: thirst, urination, and fatigue. If you let your body get used to these feelings they soon become normal for you, and then I think you are headed for trouble.

However, I also understand the dangers of insulin reactions, but with Dr. Stoney's careful instruction, I learned to keep my blood sugar as close to normal as possible. Does that mean my blood glucose level never ran high or low occasionally? Don't be ridiculous. Of course it did, and sometimes the good doctor and I, went round and round about those high blood sugars. I'm sure he wondered if I would ever get the message of good control through my thick head. Nevertheless, with his careful supervision I finally learned that control using three separate tools: insulin, exercise, and eating, which allowed me that proper balance.

I share these things with you only because I care about you, for I've seen far too many diabetics stumble and fall. And sometimes they seem so unconcerned about getting back up again. Now, it's no crime to fall, and we are all going to do this occasionally, but the winners will always be those that pick themselves up, brush themselves off, and continue again on their walk.

It takes a good doctor-patient relationship to be successful, and together you should devise a control plan that works well for you. If your doctor is not capable of that plan, then I would suggest you find a doctor that is. Remember, you need to have complete confidence, faith, and trust in your doctor, but also remember, he needs to have the same confidence, faith, and trust in you. If you will not take the responsibility for your own control, there is not much he can do for you. One more reminder: don't ever try to fool your doctor for in the end you will find, you were only fooling yourself.

I can hear parents of diabetic children and teens saying, "Do you mean you never ate anything you shouldn't have." Again, I say, don't be ridiculous; of course I did, and your child will too. But recognizing the feelings of a high blood sugar, and hating those feelings enough to take action will do more for your diabetic control then anything I know.

Mother accompanied me once more to Dr. Stoney's office, and then I was on my own. My first year was filled with monthly visits. On specified Saturday mornings I went to Hamot Hospital for a fasting blood sugar. Then, the following Monday at four o'clock I would have my checkup. That way I never missed school.

One Monday afternoon following my checkup Dr. Stoney said, "Mary, I want you to meet me at Hamot Hospital next Saturday morning."

I started to open my mouth, but he held up his hand to quiet me.

"Not to get a blood sugar," he said smiling. He knew how I hated them!

"I have two patients I want you to meet."

"Oh boy" that sounded great, especially, a visit to the hospital without getting a blood sugar.

The following Saturday morning as I waited for Dr. Stoney at the front desk, I couldn't help wondering what this was all about. Soon, Dr. Stoney appeared, and motioned for me to sit down beside him in the waiting room.

"Mary," he began, "I have two patients here who are experiencing difficulty controlling their diabetes. The sights aren't pretty, but I want you to see them, and for only one reason. I never want this to happen to you. Will you go with me to visit them?"

Well, of course I'd go. "Follow me then," he motioned.

The first room we entered was the worst. It was dark and it didn't smell very good. There was a man in bed all covered up, except for his right leg, which was only a stump wrapped in a white bandage. Dr. Stoney talked with the man, but I didn't say a word. When we stepped outside the door, he asked, "Do you want to continue or stop?"

Well certainly, I wanted to see the other patient.

"I'm not a baby you know." The next room was exactly the same thing. Another man another leg off. We walked back to the waiting room, and he and I talked for a long time.

On the bus ride home I couldn't help but think of what I had seen. If this is what happens with poor control, I'd never let it happen to me. I ran off the bus, and into the drug store to tell mother all about it.

However, she was not surprised, as Dr. Stoney had checked with her to make sure it was okay before inviting me.

Please don't get up in arms here. I hate these fears as much as you do, but I strongly believe we can turn these fears into our most valuable asset in helping us control our diabetes. And every diabetic should know exactly what can happen with uncontrolled diabetes. It certainly made a lasting impression on one little girl.

What was Dr. Stoney's motive for inviting me to the hospital to see his diabetic patients? Sometimes it is very difficult for children to fully understand everything you tell them, especially, with a new "problem" like diabetes. Warnings of high blood sugars, and what they can do will never impress them like seeing will.

Dr. Stoney's motive was not to try and frighten me to death. No, that Saturday morning the good doctor simply changed hats from physician to teacher in his unprecedented desire to help me understand just what he was trying to tell me about those high blood glucose levels.

I've often wondered what Dr. Stoney's thoughts were after that hospital trip. I'm quite sure he was filled with concern, wondering, "Will she or won't she take my instruction?"

It took time, but I finally realized that Dr. Stoney cared about me as a diabetic. All he wanted was for me to be able to enjoy a full and happy life even with my diabetes.

One event I so clearly remember after returning to grade school in January was each day's dismissal. My insulin usually peaked at that time, and I hurried, fast as I could towards home. When I got to the entrance of the Court, sweat would be dripping down my neck and forehead. I ran that last block with key in hand, until I got into the house for orange juice with sugar.

Thank goodness for Dr. Stoney. Racing home for orange juice became a thing of the past as he insisted I carry candy or sugar cubes with me at all times.

And what about my strict diet? Dr. Stoney made sure I had sufficient food as he carefully exchanged my scale and measurement existence for a wonderful new way of life called balanced eating, allowing this young diabetic girl to function naturally in a nondiabetic world.

My association with Dr. Stoney only lasted a few years. On February 1, 1959 he passed away.

He was not always fun loving and jovial like I wanted him to be. In fact, sometimes I thought he was a bit cross. However, one thing I am sure of: he was a doctor way ahead of his time in proper diabetic control. He was also the doctor that started Mary Cooper down the path of good control.

Common sense, and wisdom are inseparable in our diabetic walk. Consider the words written in the Epistle of James:

> Consider it all joy, my brethren,
> when you encounter various
> trials.
> Knowing that the testing of your
> faith produces endurance.
> And let endurance have its
> perfect result, that you may be

perfect and complete, lacking in
nothing.

But if any of you lacks wisdom,
let him ask of God, who gives to
all men generously and without
reproach, and it will be given to
him.

James 1:2–5.

Shortly after Dr. Stoney's death I was talking with another patient of his.

"You knew Dr. Stoney was a diabetic himself?" she questioned me.

"No," I replied. "If he was, he never mentioned it to me." But maybe, just maybe that was the
secret of his success.

CHAPTER 4

To My Young
Diabetic Friends

Reflecting back on my years through junior and senior high school, I have to smile. An article in the magazine "Diabetes In The News," an excellent publication, brought those times all back. In the question-and-answer section a young girl wrote:

> I'm 15 years old and have had type I insulin-dependent diabetes for the past four years. I take two injections of insulin each day and monitor my blood glucose four times a day. I'm in pretty good control, but I have some problems that I need some help on.
> I have always done my mid-day glucose test at school, in front of my girlfriends. This didn't used to be a problem. But for some reason,

this year in high school, my girlfriends object to my doing the blood test in front of them. They have started to treat me like a whole different person. I do not like this kind of treatment. How can I deal with a situation like this?

Now, I don't know how you would have answered my young friend, but the reason I am smiling is that my main objective in high school was to keep my diabetes pretty much to myself. However, that didn't mean someone close to me didn't know about my condition. It just meant I felt a little different having diabetes.

There are many books written about diabetes, but most of them are "how to" books, written by doctors or dieticians. Many of them offer excellent instruction on living with diabetes, but most authors are not capable of knowing the thoughts and feelings of a diabetic actually living with this "problem." You may, or may not agree with my thoughts regarding this diabetic walk of ours, but I want to share some of my feelings with you.

This young girl sounded a bit confused to me. I've been a diabetic for a long time, but to this day, the only people that have ever witnessed my insulin injections or blood glucose tests are family members, and I make a real effort to do them when no one is around. I've gone on vacations with friends, been to slumber parties, etc., yet there was always privacy. There was always a bathroom or a nurse's room available. Each summer I attended my church camp at the Lake Erie Bible Conference Grounds situated on Lake Erie. I was the only diabetic child at camp and I still had to take the responsibility for my control. But I loved going to camp. My urine tests and insulin injections were done in private inside the nurse's station, even at summer camp.

Remember, your diabetes should be very important to you, but as far as it being important to your friends, forget it! Don't get me wrong, it is very important that someone close to you know about your condition. But as far as trying to make your friends live in your world, I just don't think that will work.

I must confess, I am the world's worst coward. Even after living with shots and needles most of my life, I still can't stand to see someone else get an injection. In fact, when my husband's maiden aunt needed vitamin injections, I had a terrible time giving them to her. I finally turned the job over to my husband. Don't be surprised. I'm sure this is true of many diabetics. If I had been that young girl, I would have gone to the nurse's room at school to test my blood glucose.

Take my advice, don't use your diabetic condition in an attempt to attract attention to yourself. Remember, you are only one of a large number of young diabetics on this walk. Tuck the habits of good control under your arm, and open your eyes to all the wonderful things around you. Find a good hobby. I love music and spent many happy hours as a teenager playing the piano. I now have an organ. Playing gives me great enjoyment. It gets my mind off myself and it's a great stress reliever.

Once again, I hope you will understand how important it is for you to keep your eyes focused on your diabetes, but off yourself.

Along with having a loving family, I have also been blessed with many good friends. If we will look around, we can always find someone who has a "problem" much worse than ours. I will never forget the first gym class I attended in seventh grade. A girl named Audrey Adams handed the teacher a doctor's excuse. We later learned that Audrey suffered from a heart condition and could not participate in sports. I really love sports and felt a great pity for Audrey with her heart condition.

Child diabetics, as well as teenagers, often require large doses of insulin. I was no exception. I was now taking 52 units, a mixture of Regular and Protamine Zinc. Dr. Stoney worked closely with me adjusting and readjusting the insulin dosage, especially, if I was playing basketball or volleyball after school. He taught me carefully the correct way to do this adjusting myself. He knew my love for sports and he always encouraged me to participate.

Urine-testing was an important part of my life now. I loved to guess the results as I dropped the blue tablet into the test tube. I must confess my guesses were usually correct. I was adapting well to the feelings of high or low blood sugars, but that became my downfall once. I hope you will never get cocky in your diabetic control, because that can lead to trouble. After I experienced a few incorrect guesses, I soon learned to make sure rather than guess.

Our family faithfully attended Sunday School and Church services at Bethel Baptist Church in Erie, and with all the activities I was engaged in, my life was full and happy.

My adjustment in junior high school also went well. It was there I met a wonderful friend, Cynthia Hommes. Cynthia was a tall, slim brunette. She loved sports and was full of fun. We were together constantly and shared everything, including, yep, you guessed it: my diabetes. Did it make any difference to her? Absolutely not! Don't get discouraged, I'm sure you will always, somehow, know who and when to tell about your diabetic condition.

During this era I often babysat for two different neighbors: Bill and Gladyce Wallace and Bob and Ruth Mills. They were both young couples who knew about my diabetes. Never take on responsibility for someone else without informing them of your diabetes.

Both couples had two children, and whenever I babysat, they always urged me to help myself from their kitchen anytime I needed something to eat due to a low blood sugar.

Now I was a perfectly normal teenager and had quite a thing for drinking coffee back then. No one drank coffee at our house. It was over at Wallaces' house one evening I decided to take the plunge.

When you go out on a date and can order a diet coke or diet pepsi from the menu, be grateful. The only sugarless drink available to me was water, tea or coffee. Tab was the first diet pop on the market and that was still years away.

Something always fascinated me, however, when I was around people who drank coffee, especially black coffee. To a teenager back then drinking it was a real sign of maturity.

One evening, Gladyce had some leftover coffee in the coffee pot on the back burner of her stove. I heated it up and poured my first cup of real black coffee. I don't know what I expected, but the kitchen sink got most of that first mouthful. Now I was not to be undone. Drinking coffee was something I was going to learn to master. This was a sugarless drink and I struggled through that first cup.

When I told Gladyce about it, she advised me to put one of my saccharine tablets and a little milk in it.

"Get used to that first, before you try it black again," she said.

Good idea! So the following Saturday evening I walked in with my saccharine bottle. Again, I hope you will be grateful when you sprinkle a present day artificial sweetner on your food or in your drink. Saccharine was all there was when I was young and it was bitter. I finally got used to it but it was a real struggle.

Lucille Smith was another good friend. She also knew that I was a diabetic. Lucille went on to become a registered nurse after graduation. If I would have ever had trouble in school with an insulin reaction I could not handle myself, these two girls, Cynthia and Lucille knew what to do and would have helped me. Mother also informed the school principal of my condition. I would suggest you do the same. And always carry an identification card in your wallet explaining your diabetic condition.

I tend to become lazy at times. I'm twice as careful about my control when I'm alone then when my family is around. I know they will always be the first to say, "Mary, your sugar is low," without me even bothering to think about it. However, you and I are still the ones that must readily recognize the symptoms of a high or low blood sugar. Our failure to do so can be disastrous. Again I repeat, "Know YOURSELF well."

Edith and her husband Roy were now attending college at the Moody Bible Institute in Chicago, Illinois. Eleanor graduated from high school and was employed at the Telephone Company. Bill was in his senior year when I entered the tenth grade. I had many friends at school, but Cynthia and Lucille were always my special friends.

Mother was now dating a widower, Eugene Kelley. I was glad to see her go out and enjoy herself. She got me a job at Fischer & Scheller Pharmacy where she now worked. I was only fifteen, but oh, how I loved that job. Each afternoon after school I worked at the small soda fountain occasionally waiting on other customers.

The years went by rapidly. Edith and Roy graduated from college and were now serving as missionaries in Ecuador under the Wycliffe Bible Translators. Ida married Les Wells, a missionary pastor. They had a small church in Kentucky. Eleanor married Carl Tegeler, a minister with a small church in Virginia, and Bill was now a student at Moody.

After having so many brothers and sisters, all of a sudden I was alone. Mother married Eugene Kelley and for the first time in many years, got to stay home. The only thing was, there was just one left at home: Me!

Erie, Pennsylvania's main attraction is its beautiful beaches on Presque Isle. I don't think there are many Erieites who can't swim, and swimming is a favorite sport of mine.

With all the activities available to you, I again urge you to know YOURSELF well. Don't miss out on anything you want to do. Remember, it takes a great deal of energy to keep active. You can be very, very tired with either a high or low blood sugar so learn to recognize the symptoms well.

Some diabetics tend to blame uncontrolled diabetes on whatever circumstance they happen to be going through at the time. But diabetics are just as capable of adjusting to the ups and downs of life as anyone else. Don't waste your life looking for an excuse for uncontrolled diabetes. Instead, devote your energies towards developing the gumption it takes to live successfully with this "problem."

In 1954 this young diabetic girl graduated with honors from Strong Vincent High School. People back then were no different than they are today. We'll always have family and friends cheering us on, while a few scoffers tend to stand in the background wondering how we could accomplish anything in life while maintaining our good control.

A few days after graduation, Cynthia, Lucille, and myself, boarded a train at the Erie station headed for Cleveland, Ohio. There we spent three fun-filled days shopping, seeing the sights, and swimming in the hotel pool in celebration of our graduation. In a few years our paths would separate, but our friendships would never end.

The following week Cynthia and I went to the Erie Employment Office where we filled out papers and took some tests. Two days later I received a call from a woman at the employment office, advising me of a job opening at Wm. Irwin Arbuckle, a wholesale firm. It consisted of typing, which I dearly loved, along with general office work. I was scheduled for an interview the following day.

Early the next morning I found myself seated across from the business manager who conducted the interview. I told him I was a diabetic. He said, "I don't know much about that condition, but Arbuckle's needs help now!" He hired me. And I started work the following day.

I was still employed part-time at Fischer & Scheller and would not leave without giving them a week's notice. So that first week I worked at Arbuckles from 8 AM until 5 PM. Then, I worked at the pharmacy from 6 PM until 9 PM each evening. But at seventeen my energy seemed endless and I was thrilled at being a part of the work-a-day world.

Most diabetics do appreciate the many accomplishments made within our realm during the last several years which make our diabetic walk easier. However, teenagers often tell me that life was much easier back when I was young. I certainly agree!

The pressures on teenagers today are many, especially, with drug and alcohol use at an all-time high, but I'm convinced you are capable of much better things.

When you walk day in and day out, succeeding in the monotony of monitoring good diabetic control, it says a lot for you. I am sure no matter how difficult the temptations may be on you today, that you, as a diabetic, have the courage and strength to look at these enticements and turn your back on them.

Life is far too precious to waste. Many diabetic adults, including me, can now express thanks for this "problem," wondering what our lives might have been like without the stamina gained from living with diabetes.

The Bible has much to say regarding youth, and the book of Proverbs is a wealth of moral and spiritual instruction to the young. Many of the Proverbs stem from Solomon and were written to his son. But the precepts are for all youth. Consider the following words:

My son, do not forget my
teaching, But let your heart keep
my commandments;
For length of days and years of
life, and peace they will add to
you.
Do not let kindness and truth
leave you; Bind them around
your neck, Write them on the
tablet of your heart.
So you will find favor and good
repute in the sight of God and
man.
Trust in the Lord with all your
heart, and do not lean on your
own understanding.
In all your ways acknowledge
Him, and he will make your
paths straight.
Do not be wise in your own eyes;
Fear the Lord and turn away
from evil.
It will be healing to your body,
and refreshment to your bones.
Proverbs 3:1–8.

I hope you will take time to read the book of Proverbs for yourself. I am sure you will find the wisdom and admonitions given invaluable for today.

CHAPTER 5

Doctors, Doctors, Doctors

There was no application to fill out at Arbuckles, only the interview. They did however call Strong Vincent High School. I found that out when the business manager mentioned the fact that I had only missed six days of school in my three years at high school. How well I remember four of those days, because in my senior year, I came down with the three-day measles. How embarrassing!

The office in which I worked contained five people. There was a private space for Mr. Arbuckle and his son, and another office which accommodated the bookkeeping department. As I got acquainted, I kept wondering who I should tell about my "problem."

Each afternoon I worked in the bookkeeping department a few hours. The business manager also worked in this office along with the bookkeeper, Ann Eisert.

Ann was a middle-age motherly woman who had two daughters slightly younger than me. One evening while she waited for her ride to go home, I talked to her about my diabetes. Saying, "the only real danger might be an insulin reaction," (I'd never had one before that I could not handle myself) but I asked her to "please give me one of the peppermint patties I kept in my desk drawer, and make sure I ate it, if she ever saw me sweating or acting a bit confused."

I'm sure we always have a little fear when we first confide in someone new. On the way home that evening I couldn't help but worry. But my fears were groundless. Ann tucked me under her arm, like an old mother hen would her chicks. She became very interested in my "problem," and asked me many questions concerning diabetes. I never needed Ann's assistance, but knowing she was there and knew what to do to help gave me great confidence.

A few weeks later Cynthia went to work in the office of Northwest Electric. We were both delighted because Northwest Electric and Arbuckles were only a block apart. I'd been walking to work and back each morning and evening. Now I had a good friend to walk with me.

However, now that we both had jobs, Cynthia and I began thinking how sophisticated it would be to drive rather than walk to work. We searched the used car lots diligently, but without much success.

That is, until one evening, when a horn began blowing in front of our house. There sat Cynthia in a bright yellow 1948 Buick convertible. It was absolutely beautiful! A friend of her father's wanted to sell it, and he snatched it up immediately for Cynthia.

We had many good times riding in that convertible. I remember driving home from the peninsula one Saturday afternoon. A thunderstorm rolled in. She pressed the button to bring the top up, but it got stuck half way up. We got soaked, pulling, and tugging, trying to get the top the rest of the way up.

Naturally, I wanted a car of my own, and before winter, I found a used Chevrolet. I can't remember what year, but it was just perfect for me. Driving didn't allow me much exercise, and so to compensate, I joined the YWCA so I could swim several evenings each week. Cynthia, of course, joined too. Life always seems so much better when you can share it with a friend.

I was still active in my church which had a large youth group. The group met before church each Sunday evening. It was there I met another good friend, Ann McLallen. Ann had recently graduated from college and was employed in the offices of Hamot Hospital. Like Cynthia and Lucille, we are still good friends today.

However, at this point in time, mother was getting a bit frustrated with me. After Dr. Stoney's death I had not bothered to put myself in the hands of a capable doctor. She was a wise woman and knew the ground rules for good diabetic management. She went ahead and made an appointment for me with a doctor she had been impressed with during her drug store days.

The doctor was rather new in town, but I realized even before we met that our relationship would never work. He is still an excellent physician. But I was immature and kept comparing him to Dr. Stoney. After several visits he wanted me to enter a hospital so he could change my insulin to NPH, a new type that was now available. But I informed him that "I was doing just fine" and refused to go. Remember, when I mentioned that your doctor can't help you unless you are willing to help yourself. Well, I knew exactly what I was talking about. In fact, I'm sure that doctor was relieved when I did not return for another appointment.

Now mother was never one to put up with much nonsense and she gave me a limited time to choose another doctor for myself.

Dad Kelley went to Dr. Harrison Tate, a doctor mother knew and liked. Another doctor shared his office, Dr. Usher. One evening when mother had an appointment for a flu shot with Dr. Tate, I offered to drive her to his office. When we arrived Dr. Tate was out on an emergency and Dr. Usher was caring for Dr. Tate's patients as well as his own. I accompanied mother into his office and liked Dr. Usher's personality immediately. During our drive home I told mom I would call and make an appointment with Dr. Usher. I'm sure she was very relieved.

What about doctors, especially, in relationship to our diabetic control? As I continue my walk I picture them much like the coach in a basketball or football game. When that coach examines us, he or she knows exactly how well we are playing the game. Some physicians might cheer us on if they see we are

playing well. But for others, they just sadly shake
their heads.

Did you ever watch a coach sit down on the
side-lines, and hold his head between his hands when
his team is playing badly? I'm sure our doctors do exactly the same thing when they see us lax in our control. I'm also convinced that these coaches have a
pretty good idea just who is going to win in this diabetic game.

I know several Type I diabetics who have
not seen a physician in years and that bothers me.
Now your control plan might be working beautifully,
but you still need some expert coaching.

If I were shopping for a doctor, the first
qualification I'd consider would definitely include a
careful eye examination. Later on, I will share some of
my experiences dealing with eyesight, but when
changes in our diabetes take place, they can usually
first be spotted in our eyes.

If you are without a coach, I hope you will
make it your business to find one. If you are well-
controlled, he or she probably won't spend much time
with your diabetes. But having diabetes does not set
us apart from contacting other illnesses or accidents.
And I know my own diabetic walk has gone much
smoother because I have a good coach.

Dr. Usher was probably in his late fifties.
During my first appointment he smiled easily and our
personalities blended. That is very important, especially with young diabetics. I was now 19, and he listened patiently as I told him everything from Dr.
Walsh, to Dr. Stoney, and also about the doctor I
refused to go to. When I finished talking, he just

smiled. After examining me, he sat down at his desk while we again went over my entire control program.

At this particular time I was having problems early in the morning. Many mornings I would not wake up until mother spooned orange juice with sugar down my throat. That is not a simple task, especially, if you fight help occasionally, like I sometimes did.

Here again, the next time you check your blood glucose level on your Blood Glucose Monitoring Machine, remember to give it a little hug for me. When I tested my urine at bedtime, and it was negative, or blue, I knew my control was good. But how negative was negative? Are you still following me? In other words, I didn't know if it was a negative 62 blood sugar which required more food, or a negative 120 blood sugar, which only required a small snack to get me through the night. All I had to depend on was how I felt.

Dr. Usher lowered my insulin dosage, and instructed me to always make sure there was a trace of sugar in my urine at bedtime.

What tremendous insight is required each time our doctors offer instruction on our control plan. And I'm sure that responsibility weighs heavily on them.

In the Bible, the Gospel according to Luke was written by a doctor. In Colossians the Apostle Paul refers to him as:

"Luke, the beloved physician."
Colossians 4:14.

At times we get irritated with our doctor's endless instruction, and occasionally they do make mistakes. However, they are only human, and most of them would do anything they possibly can to make our diabetic walk easier for us.

CHAPTER 6

Especially For Women

Now, girls, pull your chairs a wee bit closer, and let's talk about men. This, of course, is a favorite subject of mine, and all kidding aside, every fear and thought that's ever crossed your mind regarding this subject and your diabetes has also crossed mine.

However will we handle our "problem" in dating relationships? Will it be possible to have a happy marriage with this "problem?" And then we think; "oh, if only I could run away from it now!"

Like many young women, I'd sometimes dream about my knight in shining armor coming just in the nick of time to rescue me from some terrible disaster! In that one split second we'd fall in love, but my dream sadly faded when I whispered in his ear, "I'm an insulin-dependent diabetic!" I could then picture him dropping me on my bottom end and dashing off to rescue someone else.

These fears are very common among young diabetic women. Once the mother of a teenage diabetic girl asked me how I handled those dating years? I gave her that well known answer, "Just like I'd handle a porcupine; very cautiously."

When I first began dating, like most young women I wanted to have a good time, and I especially liked boys who had a good sense of humor.

However, I soon learned to pick and choose my dates carefully, and my dating years were filled with wonderful times. Remember, you don't have to date everyone that asks you.

Mother, having raised her children alone, had one ground rule that applied to each of us. You had to be 21 before you could get married. She would not accompany any of us to the Court House and sign for us to get a marriage license.

She used to talk with her girls many times about this. In fact, we all understood that if our marriages failed due to our poor judgment or immaturity, we were all on our own. In other words, the door to home closed behind us when we married. It wasn't a swinging door. She encouraged us to date and we were more than welcome to bring our dates home. But when we married, the responsibility for that marriage rested on us.

At one time this caused a lot of friction between us, because at 20, I thought I had found Mr.

Right and was engaged to be married. But mother's rule stood firm. That romance soon faded. As I look back today, I'll always be especially grateful for mother's ground rule.

Just how does womanhood affect our diabetes? Many diabetic women do not experience any notable change, but each month approximately 48 hours before menstruation I usually had a noticeable increase in my urine sugar, and without fail, 12 to 24 hours prior to menstruation, there was always a noticeable drop. I had to pay special attention to insulin reactions at that time.

One summer in the late 1950's Ann McLallen and I attended a Bible conference at Winona Lake, Indiana. The guest soloist was George Beverly Shea. Ann knew I was a diabetic, and before I had a chance to tell her myself, mother informed her that I had to eat my meals on time.

Don't get upset if your parents ever do this. Just remember, parents tend to worry, and even if we think they overstep their bounds at times, it is something we can overlook.

That year I decided I needed a better car to drive as the Chevrolet was coughing a bit. Dad Kelley always drove Buicks, and one Saturday morning he and mother found a beautiful two-tone model for me. Only thing wrong was the price. It was a little out of my range.

Arbuckles was a nice place to work, but the pay was small, and there was no opportunity for advancement. I definitely needed more money if I intended to buy that car, so I scanned the newspaper want ads daily. Soon a job advertisement appeared in the offices of Bucyrus-Erie Company. Typing was required and the pay was excellent.

The following day I packed something to eat, and during my lunch hour from Arbuckles, applied for the job. Bucyrus-Erie was a large company. The main head-quarters were in Milwaukee, Wisconsin, while other offices and plants were located in Erie.

That afternoon I filled out my first job application, and where the health status was required, I wrote, "diabetic, (well-controlled)." A man asked me a few questions. I was given a typing test, but there was no real interview.

On Monday morning mother received the call I was hoping for. Bucyrus-Erie had indeed hired me. I was to begin work the following Monday. She phoned me at Arbuckles, relaying the news. I immediately told Mr. Arbuckle. He realized there was no future for me with his company. He also hinted about someday discontinuing the wholesale business. A year later the company closed.

The office at Bucyrus-Erie was large by my standards: 22 employees with ample room between desks and a glass enclosed office for the boss, Mr. Wheeler. My first assignment was typing parts invoices for the various machines the company sold. The billing machine I used was slightly different from a regular typewriter, however, it didn't take long to learn the procedure. Everyone in the office was exceptionally nice. The office manager was Jerry Pettit. No bill was mailed out without his approval.

That fall I celebrated my 21st birthday. Could it be possible I had actually survived ten years as a diabetic? The habits of good control were becoming so ingrained in me that I no longer felt different about having this "problem."

Twenty-one is a wonderful age. I enjoyed my work tremendously, and was now driving a nice Buick car.

I resumed dating, but many times preferred an outing with my girlfriends. We always had a good time together.

The New Year's Eve of 1959 is one I will never forget. Ann McLallen and I were planning to attend the New Year's Eve service at our church. We'd been invited to a party afterwards, given by our youth director. Ann would then spend the night at my house. That way neither one of us would be driving home alone.

The early evening was cool and misty, and after church, we went to the party with friends. However, following the party we stepped outside to find much colder temperatures and slick ice covering the streets. Our friend did not have snow tires on his car. So before starting out he put chains on his tires. It was really slippery driving, but we soon arrived at the church parking lot safely. Our friend wanted to wait until we got started, but he had a car full to take home, and we sent him on his way.

This weather did not frighten me. I love winter along with all the cold and snow it brings, and living in Northwestern Pennsylvania makes most drivers able to cope with adverse driving conditions.

My car was the only one in the icy parking lot and was parked facing a fence. I started the car. Then, after warming the motor, I put the gear shift in reverse. Even with snow tires on the car, when I put my foot on the gas pedal nothing happened. I knew better then to rev the motor, yet no matter how patiently I applied the gas, the car just would not back up, but kept sliding helplessly to one side in the icy parking lot.

Ann and I decided we were getting nowhere fast. We looked around, but the church was dark and locked tight. There wasn't a telephone booth handy, so we decided to walk up the street and see if we could telephone for help from someone's house.

Monroe Street, by the parking lot of the church, would look at home in San Francisco. We started at the bottom of the hill, and with the ice to contend with, it became a hilarious adventure.

My friend was raised in the country. She very seldom went out without boots during our long Erie winters. Being a city girl, I was not as careful. In fact, I was wearing high heels with those beautiful new pointed toes that had recently hit the shoe stores. My shoes just would not work properly on that icy uphill walk. Ann had all she could do to stay upright walking with boots. However, we persevered, slowly but surely, until reaching a house with a light shining brightly through the window.

Sitting down on the bottom porch step, I eased myself slowly up the staircase while Ann pushed the doorbell. To our dismay, no one answered. I was wearing a full length coat, so after easing myself up the steps so well, I decided to sit down on the sidewalk and dig my high heels into the ice hoping to slide myself up the hill. It worked! Soon, Ann and I were at the top of Monroe Street.

I was exhausted from laughing and struggling on the ice. It was now way past my bedtime. I'd eaten a sandwich at the party, but with all the excitement, I could feel my blood sugar level tumbling. When I get excited, it always goes down, and with long-acting insulin working overnight in my body, I could not take a chance. I ate a small peppermint pattie at the top of the hill.

We never know what kind of situations we may encounter in life. As diabetics, we must always be prepared for the unexpected.

It was much easier walking on 28th Street, and we passed a house just as a car turned into a driveway. A couple got out, and much to our surprise, it was a woman Ann knew. She graciously allowed us to use their telephone. We called our youth director, explaining our problem. In just a few minutes he appeared at the kind woman's house and drove us to my house. After all that excitement, you can be sure it didn't take Ann or me long to fall asleep that night.

Roller skating was another activity I dearly loved, and when Dad Kelley's daughter, Ruth, moved to a new apartment, she gave me her ice skates. They fit perfectly and many winter hours were spent ice skating on the bay.

Those morning insulin reactions, though stopped for a time, were now occurring again. Dr. Usher wanted me to check into Hamot Hospital to try the new NPH insulin. This time I agreed. My hospital stay lasted four days. I immediately preferred the NPH insulin because I did not have to bother mixing it.

However, it was during this hospital stay that the veins in my right arm collapsed from so many blood sugars. Now all my blood work had to be done from my left arm. It was years later a technician finally gave up on my left arm, and when I hesitatingly offered my right arm, we were both delighted when a small vein surfaced again. Now you know why I urge you to give your Blood Glucose Monitoring Machine a hug for me each time you use it. I'm engaged in a true love affair with mine.

My summer vacations were spent with friends or visiting my brothers and sisters. I loved riding the train to Chicago where Bill and his wife Ginny now lived. Bill was continuing his education, and looking forward to teaching school some day. He obtained several degrees and is now a school principal in Scottsdale, Arizona.

Advancements kept coming at Bucyrus-Erie, and when the office manager submitted his resignation, I received the promotion. This looked wonderful at first; however, I soon found out I'm a poor boss. I had a terrible time telling other people what to do.

Each time I had a conference with Mr. Wheeler, I would mention how much I disliked the position, but he just smiled and said, "You'll learn to like it." I never did. Several conferences later I informed Mr. Wheeler that I was looking for another job. He immediately hired a new office manager while I assumed the title Assistant Manager. Ah, happiness again. The new office manager was a friend I already knew from Bethel Church and we enjoyed working together.

My pal Cynthia had started to pursue her latest interest: flying. She was attending ground school classes at the Erie airport. She wanted me to take the instruction with her, but this was one interest we just could not share. I always felt a bit better with my feet planted firmly on the ground. In fact, I have a difficult time climbing more than six feet up on a ladder.

It was at this school Cynthia met another girl taking the same course, Mary Greene. But that's your name you say. Right, my sister-in-law and I share the same name. Cynthia introduced us and we soon became friends.

Mary lived in Springboro, a small town 35 miles from Erie. She then worked in the offices of the Albro Packing Company in Springboro. Mary had an older sister, Ruth, who was employed at a local bank, and two brothers, Gerald and John, who owned and operated a dairy farm in Springboro. The brothers were both pilots, and Mary had recently earned her pilot's license. The family owned a Cessna 175 Skyhawk airplane for which they rented a hangar at the Erie airport.

My first airplane flight was one summer evening with Mary, a friend of hers from Springboro, and Cynthia. Cynthia sat up front with Mary, and the four of us chatted while Mary flew the airplane. The flight was beautiful; however, I still was not all that keen on being up so high. I'm not afraid to fly; it's just not my favorite way of traveling.

It was also during this era that rumors began circulating at Bucyrus-Erie. "The billing department is going to be moved out of the Erie office and to the company headquarters in Milwaukee, Wisconsin" was the latest whisper. But there was nothing certain yet, just rumors.

The following winter Cynthia and I received an invitation from Mary Greene to come to Springboro and ice skate on their pond. It was a beautiful day, and after skating we were invited to see the new house they recently completed. It was then I met her sister Ruth, brother Gerald, and Mrs. Greene. Mary's father passed away when she was only ten. I never got to meet John. He had a date that afternoon.

It was the following spring before I finally met John. Cynthia introduced him not as John, but Willy. His name is John Willis, however, his family and close friends always call him Willy. Everyone else knows him as John. He was tall, fair complexioned, extremely polite, and of course, handsome. To say the least I was impressed.

Willy and I visited at several different functions that summer. In September of 1961 he phoned and invited me to view Niagara Falls with him from the air the following Sunday afternoon. I'd only flown that once with his sister, but how could I ever refuse an invitation like that.

The next few days I was pretty excited thinking about our date. Finally Sunday arrived. I could hardly concentrate during the morning church service, and at dinner my appetite faded. Mother reminded me: I'd better eat! "You wouldn't want to have an insulin reaction while you're flying," she said matter-of-factly.

"Oh no, that would be terrible," and thankfully I took her advice.

Wouldn't it be nice if we could take a break from this "problem" of ours every once in a while. But even if I choose to ignore it at times it still remains with me. I guess you might say we are stuck with each other, this thing called diabetes and me. And what about telling Willy about my "problem?" Well, I wouldn't want to mention it to him while he was flying the airplane. It might frighten him so badly we'd crash! Anyway, why spoil a perfectly beautiful Sunday afternoon talking about diabetes.

It was a beautiful afternoon. Willy started the motor and up we glided. The panoramic view from the front was impressive and it was smooth as glass. The fall colors looked like patchwork from the air and the view of Niagara Falls was breathtaking. He teased me a bit knowing I did not like flying all that well, but he wanted me to see just how exquisite the fall of the year looked from the air.

It was so easy to carry on a conversation with him and he was quite knowledgeable on many subjects. But all too soon our afternoon ended. In parting, he mentioned that he would call me the following week with plans for another Sunday.

It was difficult trying to get myself back out of the clouds, and down to earth again; however, on Monday morning I hit solid ground.

Mr. Wheeler called everyone into his office and lowered the boom. The billing department was indeed going to be transferred to Milwaukee, Wisconsin. Mr. Wheeler would be heading up that department and he was offering a job in Wisconsin to anyone willing to make the move.

Four people in our office were going to be transferred to other various departments within the company and the remaining employees would be laid off. He dismissed the group, except for those four names. Mine was among them. I would be transferred to the payroll department.

What a blow this was! Not only would our office group be separated, but I was totally dismayed, knowing my friends would be laid off while I still had a job.

It was two weeks before the billing department closed. I'd been transferred immediately to the payroll department and began the painstaking process of learning a new job.

The work I loved so much was gone, as well as the many friends with whom I'd shared my working days and hours. Figuring payroll was not all that exciting, but the pay was excellent. So I decided to try and make myself like the job and gave it my best.

It was a sad day when the upstairs office finally closed and the familiar faces I'd known for so long were gone.

Wouldn't it be nice if we could just shut out all the unpleasant experiences of life? However, that would not necessarily guarantee our happiness anymore than picturing how wonderful our lives might have been without diabetes. Living without our "problem" would not necessarily guarantee our happiness. In fact, there is something very special about people who have "problems" and are able to live with them.

We also tend to forget that everyone has a handicap of some kind. The further I walk the more grateful I've become that my "problem" is only diabetes.

On Tuesday evening the telephone rang. It was the voice I wanted to hear inviting me out the following Sunday. He would meet me at church and then we would go out to dinner. It is very difficult for farm boys when it comes to dating, especially if their date lives an hour's drive from them. But Willy and Gerald had a nice arrangement. They took turns having a Sunday night off from chores.

We spent a lovely afternoon together. That night I accompanied him home and watched while he did chores. I think Greenes' barn was the first dairy barn I was ever in. I was really becoming impressed with this farmer and this new world called "farming."

Our dating continued and by this time Willy had gained mother's full approval. She really liked him. I must say this was one of the first times mother and daughter agreed about men.

Reverend Robert Gilbert was the pastor at Bethel Church while we were dating. He had grown up on a farm in Indiana and knew all about the rigors of farm life.

But this was my first opportunity to witness two farmers, one now turned preacher, talking together. It is like nothing else exists except their conversation. Its really tickled me over the years as I've watched this bond form time after time between farmers.

My job at Bucyrus-Erie was no longer unpleasant and I began making new friends. The 12th Street offices closed and our office was moved to the plant at 15th and Raspberry Streets.

In life, adjustments are sometimes difficult as adjusting to our diabetes is sometimes difficult for many of us. But don't despair, just give it some time. Dr. Snider's friend, mentioned in the preface, who was having a difficult time adjusting to the insulin injections, is a real pro at it now. He is doing beautifully.

I take my hat off to him, because I think it is far more difficult adjusting to diabetes after you have spent most of your life free from it, then it is adjusting from childhood.

During November, Willy, his sister, Mary, and I made plans to fly to New Jersey to visit friends of the Greene family. I knew I had to tell him about my "problem." So one day I just blurted it out! Much to my surprise it didn't bother him. As I got to know him better, I realized there wasn't much he was afraid of, including diabetes.

The weekend in New Jersey was great. We left early Saturday morning and arrived home before dark on Sunday. The people were warm and friendly. Saturday evening they drove us into New York City to see the sights. At Rockefeller Center we gazed at the huge Christmas tree and watched the ice skaters. The city reminded me much of a fairy tale world with all the trimmings.

At Christmas I was invited to Greenes for dinner. Willy's Aunt Marge and Uncle Elmer were there. Uncle Elmer kept us smiling and laughing most of the afternoon.

As winter progressed we occasionally visited farms whose dairy barn had a pipeline milker installed. This is a line that carries milk from the cow directly to a bulk tank. Gerald and Willy were going to install one in their barn and Willy was checking things out.

The arrival of spring brought with it an

increased work load for my farm boy, who had now taken on all appearances as my knight in shining armor.

Summer arrived and one Sunday afternoon in July Cynthia went flying with us. She was still determined to get her pilot's license. I offered to sit in the back while Willy instructed her on what is called "touch and go landings." Incidentally, that's exactly what they were. If I could have crawled out I would have. Touching down on the runway, we would glide across, then go back up in the air only to repeat the entire process again. Now one or two of these would have been fine, however, we continued for an hour or more. But what are friends for anyway.

In August Willy proposed. I knew without a doubt that he was the man I wanted to spend the rest of my life with. We set the wedding date for October and began planning the happy occasion.

Approximately two weeks before our wedding Willy was talking with a man from Springboro. He asked about me, and in the course of their conversation, Willy mentioned the fact that I was a diabetic. Whereupon, the man just shook his head sadly saying, "Diabetics are tired all the time. Are you sure you want to marry a diabetic?" It so happened that this man was related to two diabetics.

When Willy recalled the conversation to me, I could see he was troubled by the man's remark. I was sad and hurt. Sad because I loved him so dearly, and hurt that some diabetics have given you and me such a bad name. However, this was something I could not interfere with. He alone had to decide whether he wanted to marry a diabetic or not.

Of course, you already know his decision. He was not afraid. And on the second Saturday of October in 1962 we were married, pledging ourselves to each other before God.

It had now been fifteen years since the discovery of my diabetes, and had I listened to certain individuals whom I choose to call diabetic soothsayers, I probably would have drowned in self pity. According to them, I had only five years to spend with this man I had chosen to marry.

CHAPTER 7

Marriage and Me, or Marriage and I

Before writing this chapter, I asked my husband how he would describe me to strangers? One word immediately tumbled from his lips. "Stubborn!" Realizing I'd left myself wide open, I proceeded, "And just how would you describe yourself?" "Oh, I'm meek and mild," I couldn't help interrupting, "Like when I say jump! You say, how high dear?" "Exactly," he replied. I burst out laughing while my husband grinned, saying, "I think that describes me perfectly."

However, my description of the John Greene I know is a bit different from his. I think the words, "fiercely independent," describe him best, and his friends will tell you, "That's putting it mildly."

How in the world did these two very different, and obstinate personalities ever make it in marriage alone, without the added frustration of diabetes?

When I admonished young diabetics to know THEMSELVES well, it is also the best advice I can offer any diabetic, man or woman, contemplating marriage. When I repeat advice, it is simply because I have found it to be so extremely important as I follow my own diabetic walk, and knowing MYSELF well precedes everything else.

Your partner expects you to be an independent individual, and Webster's Dictionary defines the word independent as: "free from the influence, control, or determination of another." In other words, can you stand on your own two feet, especially, in relation to your diabetes?

Please, don't ever present yourself as a helpless, weak waif, needing a partner's protection because life dealt you this pitiful blow called diabetes. I've witnessed a few individuals with that attitude, and frankly it turns my stomach. Your husband or wife to be does not deserve the extra burden of an uncontrolled diabetic for a life's mate.

Nevertheless, after a brief honeymoon, this new husband and wife team began learning what married life was all about. We soon discovered that these two individuals, now one, didn't always think alike. This was frustrating! But rather than trying to control each other, and force our separate opinions down each other's throat, we simply learned to respect each other's opinion even though it might not always agree with our own.

Control is essential in our diabetic walk,

but not in regard to our relationships with one another, especially in marriage.

We moved into a small house one-quarter mile from the farm. I continued working at Bucyrus-Erie. It increased my work day from eight to ten hours because of the extra miles I was driving, and changes in my diabetic control were now essential to compensate for this.

I no longer sat down to a dinner already prepared for me after work. It was now my responsibility to prepare the meal myself, and feed a hungry husband whose dinner time was much later than mine.

How do we deal with situations that are not always ideal for our diabetes? With sound, practical judgements, better known as good, old common sense.

I'm certain you realize that when meals are going to be delayed for an insulin-dependent diabetic, it's always important for that person to eat something to keep his or her blood glucose level on an even keel. If delayed meals don't seem to bother you, check your blood glucose level, it might be running a bit high.

Shortly after our wedding, my husband and I were honored at a party given by his cousins at the local grange hall. Being a real city girl, I never dreamed what these friends and relatives were planning.

After the event they followed us home, and before long I found myself seated in a wheelbarrow being pushed by my husband through the small town of Springboro. I must admit it was a lot of fun, and a real initiation to country living.

One morning at work a vivacious young woman walked up to my desk. "Are you Mary Greene?" she inquired. I nodded my head "yes."

"I just started working in the office downstairs a few days ago," she began. "I'm also a diabetic. When I applied for this job I was frightened; it's my first job. I thought there might be a problem because of my diabetes, and at my interview they questioned my condition. They also told me they had a diabetic woman working for them who was an excellent employee. I just wanted to meet you, and thank you, for I'm sure you helped me get this job."

Oh what a wonderful compliment that was to this diabetic. But what an admonition! Be very careful how you live with this "problem." Your reputation could make or break the diabetic walking behind you.

Of course, we became friends immediately. I have a very special relationship with my diabetic friends. Sometimes we get to feeling so "all alone" in this diabetic world of ours, and finding a friend who has the same "problem" can often make our diabetic walk more enjoyable.

My new friend had only been a diabetic a short time and was already concerned about her future. She had a steady boyfriend, and when she conveyed stories about his reaction to some of her insulin reactions I'd just burst out laughing. I really thought she might frighten the poor boy to death. She had a wonderful sense of humor, yet I think she added just a wee bit on to her stories.

But what about these insulin reactions? One evening a doctor spoke at an Erie County Diabetes Association meeting. He said; "If you have never had an insulin reaction you are not well controlled." And I heartily agree. What did he mean?

There is a fine line between normal and low blood sugars. Very few insulin-dependent diabetics can walk this line perfectly without leaning a wee bit under at times. On the other hand, I remember another diabetic friend who was also a type I, and had never experienced an insulin reaction. I really thought that was quite strange, and later in life when she suffered a complication, I realized her fine line probably always lapsed towards the high blood glucose level side.

Don't get me wrong, insulin reactions will not prevent complications. We must also be very careful about these insulin reactions. However, my own diabetic walk has been much safer because I choose to live on the normal to low blood sugar side of the line.

What symptoms do you associate with a low blood sugar? This depends somewhat on the type of insulin you take. I think I've experienced every known symptom, plus a few more just for good measure. We should all readily recognize the symptoms, which listed in diabetic publications will read: Hunger, anxiety, headache, pounding heart, heavy perspiration, racing pulse, trembling, nausea, and fainting.

However, let's talk about them in a language we can better understand. Of course, we should all know the most common symptoms which are; tiredness, extreme weakness, and perspiration. But what are some of the others?

When I'm working at something rather strenuous and notice myself slowing down, that's a cause for concern. If I begin yawning frequently, that can also mean trouble. When anxious feelings suddenly grow out of proportion, I immediately check my blood glucose level. Occasionally, I will notice myself slightly jerking, and hunger is rarely a symptom for me as I'm usually not hungry. Sometimes I'll experience a numbness around my face and lips, as well as a numbness in my right or left hand. When I'm reading or watching television and notice a blurriness of vision, I immediately check it out. A headache, especially when I wake up with one in the morning can mean a low blood sugar, and a change in personality like extreme excitement, or when I become just plain irritable. (Good thing I have diabetes to blame that one on). And the last one I can think of is the inability to urinate.

If we could talk together, I'm sure you would have symptoms I've never experienced, and likewise, you've probably never experienced some of mine.

I'm pretty good at recognizing low blood sugars, but no matter how experienced I think I am, they still tend to sneak up on me at times, and I must always be on guard.

But don't despair; walking this diabetic path should become a real challenge to you, and the longer you walk diligently the easier it becomes.

One very necessary requirement for a healthy marriage, and a pleasurable diabetic walk is a good sense of humor. Most of all, don't be afraid to laugh at yourself. I tend to feel a bit sorry for men and women who will never get to experience marriage to a diabetic. I really think they miss out on a lot of excitement! My husband will testify to that. He could certainly write a comedy on the many humorous experiences we've shared together.

A perfect marriage does not describe ours. In fact, I'm a little afraid of a perfect marriage. But a happy marriage, that sounds like ours. Don't be afraid of this wonderful relationship, just keep yourself in shape so you will be able to enjoy it. Statistics show the divorce rate among insulin-dependent diabetics and their spouses to be extremely high.

My husband and I took a few days off work in November, enjoying a short vacation. Among other points of interest, we stopped to visit my former boss, Mr. Wheeler in Milwaukee, Wisconsin. Willy and I were now weighing the possibility of buying the farm from Gerald. However, Mr. Wheeler urged him to buy a dairy farm in Wisconsin so I could come back to work for him.

The job offer was very attractive, and I would have loved working for Mr. Wheeler again, but I had someone else's wishes to consider now.

We arrived back in Erie just in time for my scheduled appointment with Dr. Usher. I'd told him all about Willy, and now I wanted them to meet. After my examination we spent over an hour talking. I felt sorry for his other patients, but Dr. Usher was in no hurry. I knew he was impressed with my husband.

One afternoon Reverend Gilbert and Willy were talking, and Reverend Gilbert said, "I'm so sorry my children were not raised on a farm. The responsibility of caring for livestock would have been just what the boys needed. If they woke up in the morning with a headache, or stomach-ache, they couldn't call the barn, saying: I'm sick today, I won't be coming in. They would have to get out of bed, and take care of the animals anyway." I was soon going to learn exactly what he was talking about.

Our first Thanksgiving together was spent at Gladys and Wally's house. The night before, Willy's mother brought me some carrots and beets from her garden to take along to my family. I cooked some for dinner that evening, and they were delicious! How could these vegetables taste so good? I'd had carrots and beets many times before, but none that ever tasted like this! It was, admittedly, my first taste of fresh, dug garden vegetables. I'll never forget that taste.

My entire family was at that Thanksgiving dinner. I still remember my young nephew, Jim, telling his new uncle that they were all afraid Aunt Mary was going to be an old maid. Seems like he'd rescued me just in the nick of time! However, by 3:30 that afternoon we had to leave so my husband could get back for evening chores. I then recalled what Reverend Gilbert had said. Yes, I was slowly learning about this new life called "farming."

Did you think the title of this chapter a wee bit strange? Marriage and Me, or Marriage and I? Oh, those me's and I's can cause so much trouble, not only in a diabetic's marriage, but in any marriage. And over the years we've learned that when we remove the 'Me' and the 'I' from our marriage it works beautifully.

I have been especially blessed with a husband that not only cares about me, but also cares about my "problem." I know this is not always true in diabetic marriages. And I consider myself most fortunate. Over the years when problems with my diabetes have occasionally surfaced, my knight-in-shining armor does not turn his back on me saying, "that's your "problem," you handle it!" No, he gently encircles me

in his arms and says: "This is our "problem" now.
We'll handle it."

Consider with me the "more excellent
way," as described in Corinthians:

> If I speak with the tongues of
> men and of angels, but do not
> have love, I have become a noisy
> gong or a clanging cymbal.
>
> And if I have the gift of prophecy,
> and know all mysteries and all
> knowledge and if I have all faith,
> so as to remove mountains, but
> do not have love, I am nothing.
>
> And if I give all my possessions
> to feed the poor, and if I deliver
> my body to be burned, but do not
> have love, it profits me nothing.
>
> Love is patient, love is kind, and
> is not jealous; love does not brag
> and is not arrogant,
>
> does not act unbecomingly; it
> does not seek its own, is not
> provoked, does not take into
> account a wrong suffered,
>
> does not rejoice in
> unrighteousness, but rejoices
> with the truth.
>
> bears all things, believes all
> things, hopes all things, endures
> all things
>
> Love never fails; but if there are
> gifts of prophecy, they will be
> done away; if there are tongues,
> they will cease; if there is

knowledge, it will be done away.

For we know in part, and we
prophesy in part;
But when the perfect comes, the
partial will be done away.

When I was a child, I used to
speak as a child, think as a child,
reason as a child; when I became
a man, I put away childish
things.

For now we see in a mirror dimly,
but then face to face; now I know
in part, but then I shall know
fully just as I also have been
fully known.

But now abide faith, hope, love,
these three; but the greatest of
these is love.

I Corinthians 13.

CHAPTER 8

A Time for Joy

In the spring of 1963, after carefully weighing all the possibilities, my husband and I purchased Gerald's half-interest in the farm. This was a tremendous decision for us to undertake, but we were young and energetic.

The initial farm consisted of 300 acres in four separate pieces. 100 acres of this land included the barn and house where we live, along with another 100 acres two miles east of the home farm. This land also afforded a barn and house. Willy's maiden aunt lived in the house, and the barn provided winter protection for our replacement cattle.

Also included was another piece of land one mile northwest of the home farm. It had an existing barn with 20 acres of land which provided summer pasture for our heifers, and finally an additional 80 acres of land located a mile northwest of the home farm.

Along with the land we purchased 40 head of Holstein milk cows, including 40 replacement heifers and calves, and the existing machinery on the farm at that time.

I continued working at Bucyrus-Erie, and with winter's icy blast only a memory now, I delighted in driving to work on those beautiful spring mornings.

In June of that year Dr. Usher confirmed what I already suspected: a third Greene would be arriving to help us manage the newly purchased farm. My due date was the second week in January of 1964.

Diabetic women have not always shared the favorable results in pregnancy that are common today, and in years past physicians were striving to make this journey safe for all diabetic women. The progress since then has been astounding. Diabetic women contemplating pregnancy are living in a great age. We've come a long way since the discovery of my diabetes in the 1940's. With the proper use of the Blood Glucose Monitoring Machine, diabetic women today need not fear pregnancy.

Quite unexpectantly, however, I began noticing some very different circumstances in regard to my diabetic management. It was becoming increasingly difficult for me to determine a low blood sugar: No weakness, no sweating, no inability to concentrate, none of the usual symptoms which had previously made insulin reactions so easy to recognize.

In fact, the low blood sugars I was now experiencing had few symptoms. I'd catch my head weaving. If I had not acknowledged this, and slipped something sweet into my mouth, I hate to think what might have happened.

My desk at Bucyrus-Erie was beside David Alexander's. David was a very pleasant, considerate young man. Without my asking for help, David realized my plight. Many times when my head started to droop he would dash for a bottle of pop or a cup of sugar-sweetened coffee for me to drink.

This was my first experience needing outside help to correct a low blood sugar during daylight hours. That fall it would be 16 years I'd taken care of this kind of problem myself. My stubborn nature just did not know quite how to react to David's kindness.

After one particularly bad afternoon in which David again came to my rescue, I reconstructed the entire event to my husband that evening. I expected him to sympathize with me on my inability to recognize the insulin reaction; however, he ignored my request for sympathy, saying, "Please thank David for me."

Mrs. Peg Hohler was the nurse at Bucyrus-Erie at that time. Her youngest daughter, Patty, and I had been friends in school. Of course, Mrs. Hohler knew about my diabetes. In fact, she had instructed David on just what he should do. When I realized these two friends were making it their business to look out for me my pride crumbled. How fortunate I was to know people like Mrs. Hohler and David Alexander.

Dr. Usher was not overly concerned about these insulin reactions. He was under the opinion that they would only exist a short time during my pregnancy. He and I had already discussed the great distance I was driving. We both agreed that I should find an obstetrician, and a diabetic physician closer to home that would work together.

I intended to find this team of doctors in Meadville, a town which was only a 30 minute drive from Springboro. I intended to submit my resignation to Bucyrus-Erie the middle of July, working until the end of that month to help cover for vacation time, after which, I would then become a full time farm wife.

It's always pleasant to have a day off, and on the Fourth of July while preparing breakfast I anticipated my day. Willy had finished the morning chores, and while we ate breakfast together, he ran off a list of jobs he hoped to accomplish that day. He had two college-age boys working for him that summer, but they had the day off. However, with the sun shining brightly baling hay took precedence over everything else.

As he hurried out the door, he invited me to come and have lunch with them at the farm. His mother was an excellent cook, and she often fed the farm employees. If I could have only forseen the happenings of that day, I would have run up the road fast as I could to have lunch with them.

However, I was involved in my own projects which included washing clothes, and mowing the lawn. Willy kissed me goodbye, and said he would stop later on that day, probably before evening chores.

After washing clothes, I proceeded to straighten up the house a bit. I remember being hampered by a slight headache. I tested my urine, and it was negative. It was almost noon, so rather than eat a snack to bring up my blood glucose level I sat down and ate lunch.

It's hard to remember what I ate that afternoon, but I do remember becoming very tired. In fact, I rinsed my lunch dishes, and piled them on the drainboard by the kitchen sink which is something I never do.

Actually, I was way ahead of schedule, and thought I'd certainly have more pep to mow the lawn if I took a short afternoon nap. I remember locking the back door before laying down on the couch. I was not well acquainted with this area yet, and after living in the city so long, I just presumed that everybody locked their doors in the country. I never once thought about a low blood sugar, especially after eating lunch, and thought I'd now found the perfect time to enjoy this nap.

As the day progressed my husband became increasingly concerned because he had not seen me outside mowing the lawn or feeding the heifers, which was a new project I'd taken on. They were in a pasture close to our house.

When Willy finished bailing hay, he raced home and tried to open the back door; however, it was locked tight. He ran around to the front porch, but I'd also latched the front screen door. He then saw me stretched out on the living room couch.

Realizing something was wrong, he worked frantically breaking in a cellar window. When he reached me, he said the couch was soaked in sweat, and I was cold and clammy from an insulin reaction.

He ran to the kitchen, but in his excitement forgot to put the sugar in liquid. He took a spoonful of sugar, and slowly eased it into my mouth.

Of course, I choked. He said, "You actually turned blue." Then, he held me upright, praying I would not choke to death. When the choking finally subsided, he ran to the telephone and summoned his mother.

In a matter of minutes she was at our house with the station wagon. He carried me outside, carefully placing me in the station wagon. By this time, according to him, "My body was stiff as a board." My mother-in-law held my head up, while my husband broke all speed limits getting us to Meadville.

My sister-in-law, Mary, had the presence of mind to phone the emergency room at City Hospital. She told them the problem, and about what time we should be arriving. When they asked which doctor, she requested a doctor my mother- in-law was going to at the time.

According to my husband they did not treat me in the emergency room, but admitted me immediately to a private room. He remembers them starting an intravenous feeding of 5% glucose, but he can't remember anything else.

It was now after 5:00 PM, and there were evening chores to be done. But Willy knew he could count on Mary to get the cows milked.

While my husband and mother-in-law waited, the doctor was close at hand carefully analysing my condition, and he seemed increasingly puzzled when I did not respond to the treatment.

Willy went into the Men's room to wash his hands. Did you ever see a farmer after working in a hayfield all day? Well, my husband was no exception. When he walked back to the room the doctor was now quite concerned.

As the doctor and Willy talked, Willy

mentioned notifying my mother. The doctor responded by saying, "By all means, get her mother. We don't know which way this case is going."

My husband reached into his pocket for some change to use in the pay phone, but his pockets were empty. He didn't even have his wallet or driver's license with him. He hoped maybe his mother had some money with her; however, she had left the house so quickly when he called that she neglected to pick up her purse.

A nurse on duty was Margaret Hamilton, a close neighbor of my in-laws. How grateful my husband was to see Margaret. He quickly borrowed some change from her to use in the telephone, along with enough cash to buy gas. While racing towards Meadville, he noticed the gas gauge hovering near empty.

With my husband headed towards Erie, my mother-in-law sat with me, hoping I would soon respond.

Mother was ready when Willy reached her house. They did not waste any time getting back to the Meadville hospital. But my mother-in-law sadly informed them that I had not made any progress.

Mary came to take her mother home, and brought her brother a change of clothes. When they left, mother and Willy sat quietly, silently praying for some response from me.

When the hands of the clock reached midnight, mother urged Willy to go home and try to get some sleep. She promised she would call him immediately if my condition changed. He left the hospital that night, weighed down, with little assurance he would ever see me alive again. This strong, determined man, who had not been afraid to marry the diabetic woman he loved, was now surely being sorely tried.

Mother moved close to my bed, and held onto the hand that was free from the intravenous. She was no stranger to troubles in her life, and her supreme faith in God had always pulled her through before. I'm sure that evening she once again committed her daughter to Him, knowing He would work his perfect will in my life.

Her thoughts drifted back to the November evening in 1947, when she first sat by the bedside of her young daughter at Saint Vincent's Hospital in Erie. That night she had been stunned by the diagnosis of diabetes, not knowing how it would affect my young life, and now, almost sixteen years later she was again sitting with the young woman, who, until now, had fared quite well with that diabetic diagnosis. After a while she settled back, and sipped some hot tea the nurse brought her. Together they hoped for some response.

Morning dawned, and mother was slightly encouraged because I had started to move a bit.

Dr. Fred Ewing, a Meadville obstetrician had been called in on my case. The big question was how this insulin reaction was affecting the new life within me. Dr. Ewing was quite sure my liver would supply the necessary sugar to the baby; however, he had never been involved in an insulin reaction of such duration.

Shortly after eight o'clock that morning my husband telephoned Bucyrus-Erie, and told my boss what had happened. In a sorrowful voice Willy said, "If Mary recovers, I can't allow her to keep working."

Of course, my boss understood.

"Please keep us informed, we are all pulling for her," he replied.

Willy rushed back to the hospital after finishing morning chores and giving the boys some work to do. Farming never stops! Mother went to the snack shop for breakfast. Then, Willy noticed I was moving just a bit more.

When mother returned, I could hear her voice along with my husband's. They were talking to someone. Why was mother here, and who was my husband talking to? Where was I anyway? They seemed so concerned! I could move my hands and feet. Oh, how I wanted to talk to them, to tell them I was all right.

This is probably the most frustrating state of the temporarily deprived consciousness of a severe insulin reaction. Your response comes back so slowly. I opened my eyes and could see them, but I could not talk. I realized I was in a hospital when I saw the intravenous feeding.

"Oh, no." I finally concluded what had happened. And was I uncomfortable. I had to urinate, but I couldn't get that message across to anyone.

Finally, shortly after eleven o'clock that morning everything came together. My first words were, "Willy, I have to go to the bathroom."

Tears of joy spilled down their cheeks as the nurse pulled the bedpan from the cabinet. It was difficult for me to believe I'd been unconscious that long.

What a headache I had, yet the worry and concern I'd caused my family hurt me more. My hus-

band was so gracious. He realized I'd eaten before laying down because of the dishes I'd left on the
drainboard.

"It's not like Mary to leave dishes undone," he said.

Whatever was happening with this pregnancy?

A nurse immediately brought me a huge
breakfast. She urged me to eat everything. That was
impossible. I ate what I could, and then they removed
the intravenous feeding.

After the doctor examined me I was moved
into a 2-bed room. The doctor did not want to release
me immediately, and chose to hospitalize me a few
days, so they could observe these insulin reactions.

Naturally, I had to rejoice with my family
and the nurses, as they recalled the preceeding 24
hours to me. They were so exuberant, and once again I
was reminded of the wonderful, loving, caring family
I've been blessed with.

Willy hugged me tenderly, and started for
home. I hoped the farm work would not fall behind
schedule due to this episode in our lives. Needless to
say, Willy was anxious to tell his family the good news
and also inform our friends.

A short time later Gladys and Wally
walked into my hospital room. Mother had informed
my brothers and sisters about the insulin reaction
while she was waiting for Willy that evening, and now
they shared in my joyful recovery. After visiting, they
took mother with them and started for home.

Now alone, I laid my head back on the pil-
low and stretched my hands over my stomach. A tear
trickled down my cheek as I wondered what effect this

insulin reaction might have on the tiny life within me.

My thoughts were interrupted, however, when a man sporting a huge smile walked up to my bed. "I'm Dr. Fred Ewing," he introduced himself. Right away I recognized the name. This was the obstetrician they had called in.

Jokingly, he said, "I'm very glad to meet you. For a while last night I wasn't sure I'd ever get the chance." I burst out laughing while he chuckled, appreciating his sense of humor. But when the laughter subsided, he already knew the question that was troubling me: How would this insulin reaction affect the baby?

His reply was the same as he had given to my family. The liver acts as a protector, and should have supplied the baby with the necessary sugar. Immediately the words:

> For thou didst form my inward
> parts, thou didst weave me in
> my Mother's womb.
> I will give thanks to thee, for I
> am fearfully and wonderfully
> made; Wonderful are thy works.
> Psalm 139:13,14.

came to mind. How miraculous it was that the Lord had already provided the necessary protection to keep this baby from danger.

The question of why these insulin reactions were occurring so frequently, and why such a severe one had occurred in the first trimester of my pregnancy was indeed puzzling.

High blood glucose levels are sometimes detected in non-diabetic women during pregnancy. Usually, diabetic women must be very careful of high blood glucose levels, especially, in the first trimester of pregnancy. Could it be possible my pancreas was somehow producing insulin during these first months of pregnancy? That seemed to be the conclusion now drawn by everyone.

When Dr. Ewing left, I realized that I did not need to search for an obstetrician, or a diabetic physician to accompany me through this pregnancy. We had in fact already met, quite unexpectedly!

Before becoming pregnant I had few qualms about delivering a perfectly healthy child. I was a well controlled diabetic and a very healthy woman. However, after this insulin reaction, doubts started to creep in. How grateful I was for the comfort found in my Bible.

This was the third time I'd been admitted to a hospital. The first was when they discovered my diabetes. The second was for an insulin change, and now this time for an insulin reaction. How I hoped my next hospital stay would conclude with the delivery of a healthy baby.

Shortly before dark, a tall, lean figure strode into my hospital room. How grateful I was to see him. It had been an exceptionally long day for him. Now, after evening chores, he'd driven back to see me. How tired he looked as he nestled close to me. As we talked, he again recounted the happenings of the previous day. How worried he had been, and now, how grateful he was. It was then I realized, that with him beside me, everything would be all right.

Later that evening a nurse rubbed my back. Boy, I could really get spoiled with this kind of treatment. It relaxed me and I slept soundly until morning.

A new day dawned, sunny and bright. It made me long to be home helping my husband. Could it be possible I was just a little homesick? To help pass the time I spent hours walking the hospital corridors, visiting with other patients, but just before dark each evening, my favorite visitor appeared.

He would recount everything that happened on the farm that day. The 10 acres of kraut cabbage were finally set and all the first crop hay was in the barn. I thought for sure I was missing out on everything, but he assured me there would still be plenty of work when I got home.

Willy and the college boys moved our furniture from the little house to the new farm house. His mother would be staying a few days to help me get orientated.

The following Sunday I was released from the hospital. My husband arrived to take me home, knowing I longed to stop for one last look at the little house where we first set up housekeeping. But when we walked inside, it didn't look the same with all the furniture gone, and I realized I had to say goodbye to that lovely first house we shared together, and hello to a new and exciting life awaiting me.

My first evening meal on the farm was surrounded by quite a different language then I'd ever heard spoken before. Some of Willy's family were eating with us. They talked about cows freshening, cows coming in heat. They used words like grist, stanchion, pulsator . . . these words sounded like Greek to me.

What in the world were they talking about?

Later that evening, my farm teacher and I went over some of the new terms I'd heard. I never realized that this farm profession had a language all its own.

As my mother-in-law patiently assisted me, each day on the farm seemed just a little different. Our only set pattern occurred each afternoon when we walked out in the pasture, and brought the cows into the barn. Each cow had a separate stanchion . . . . you can see I learned the meaning of that word. We would grain the cows, and feed the small calves. However, our most helpful task was running errands.

Any time a replacement part was needed, or some supply exhausted, we hurried to pick it up at whatever store or mill sold it. I was very careful about low blood sugars, especially while driving, and I ate small snacks often.

In late July Willy harvested a truck load of wheat and sold it to the Westford Mill. He had many jobs that day, and more wheat to combine, so I offered to drive the big truck to Westford to deliver the wheat.

Incidentally, I had no idea where Westford was or even how to drive that big truck. It was a 1950 Ford with the gear shift on the floor. I'd only driven automatic vehicles before. But Willy was game. He went around our circular driveway a couple of times with me, teaching me how to shift the truck. When my driving lesson was finished, I called my mother-in-law who was more than willing to accompany me to the mill.

She drove up to the farm, and the two of us started out. It was a bit different driving that big truck on the highway, but it was fun. After arriving at the mill a man unloaded our wheat. We made it back home safe and sound, while I claimed a new title: experienced truck driver.

Bob Thompson was one of the boys working for us that summer. He was attending college at Slippery Rock. One morning Bob's mother, Ann Thompson, stopped to visit. How grateful I was that Ann took time to reach out to me. However, there soon became a very special drawing attraction between us known as diabetes.

That's right, it seems hard to believe but my very first friend in the small town of Springboro was also a diabetic. Of course, we became good friends and I appreciated Ann's friendship. She also offered me advice on my new job as a farmer's wife. I needed all the help I could get with that position.

Besides keeping house and running errands, I continued walking down the lane for the cows at chore time. These cows were pretty well trained. Many times I could get them into the barn and fastened up by myself. Graining them and feeding the calves were no problem for me. After watching my husband milk, I thought perhaps I'd like to try it sometime. I didn't know much about cows. The pipeline he plugged the milker into was made of glass. It was simple to tell when the cow was finished milking. Occasionally, I'd wash a cow's teats before Willy slipped the milker on and once in a while I'd take the milker off for him.

How I loved this active life on the farm. Without even realizing it, I was exercising constantly.

My next important job was driving tractor while the boys loaded second crop hay on the wagon. The tractor was a 1955 Ford, I found driving it a bit more difficult then driving the big standard shift truck.

The hayfield also had a few slopes and inclines to deal with. It became quite a challenge to stop the tractor on one of these, while the boys picked the hay up off the ground, and stacked it neatly on the wagon.

Then, I had to ease the tractor up the grade, trying not to topple the stacked hay or the boy who was standing on the wagon. That demanding task took some patient effort on my part, but I persevered. How proud I was when I finally drove my first loaded wagon to the barn without any trouble.

Consequently, farming became as great a challenge to me as my diabetes has been. I've never been one to run from a challenge. And my new life as a farmer's wife offered me a demanding profession with a lifestyle I could easily enjoy.

When I think back to the old days of farming, they often remind me of the old days with my diabetes. Today, many wonderful advancements have been made in both fields. We no longer bale hay on the ground, but use a baler which kicks the hay directly into a wagon pulled behind it. The hay bales need only be handled when we unload them into the hay mow. We also use a large round baler which eliminates all hand labor. It only requires a machine operator to get the hay into the proper storage and then to the animals.

Likewise, with our diabetes, the ridged scale and measurement existence of insulin-dependent diabetics should be a thing of the past. All diabetics should be able to enjoy eating in restaurants today, and carefully adjusting our insulin to meet our daily food and exercise requirements, releases us from the past slavery that once dominated us.

Every three weeks during my pregnancy I was carefully examined by my obstetrician and once a month I was checked by the physician caring for my diabetes.

Large babies are usually born to diabetic mothers. Knowing this, I was EXTRA careful about my eating, as I sought to provide the baby with all the necessary nutrients without overdoing it. And my weight gain stayed perfectly normal.

I always referred to my cargo as baby John. In fact, we never picked a girl's name. I told my husband many times I just knew this baby was going to be a boy.

September came and the cabbage began to ripen. Most of the crop was contracted to the Albro Packing Company in Springboro. My husband's family often talked about cutting cabbage. I couldn't wait to try my luck at it.

It was late September when the cabbage was ready. Once again my teacher and I headed for the cabbage field. Kraut cabbage is a bit different from the cabbage you purchase at your grocery store. Most heads weighed from 17 to 20 pounds. It took a sharp, quick hand to pierce the cabbage stump and send the knife on through it.

After trying it, I realized cutting cabbage wasn't going to be all that simple. But the exercise was what I was after, so I gave it my best. Sometimes I'd get the knife half-way through the thick stump and it would stop. Then, I sawed back and forth until the knife made it all the way through.

The first row was easy. I just pushed the

huge leaves back, and cut through the core leaving the cabbage lay. The next three rows had to be cut and tossed into the original row. We always cut eight rows at a time throwing four rows into one. That left plenty of room to drive a truck or wagon between the rows.

However, loading cabbage was quite a different matter. The racks on the truck were high. I'd take a pitchfork, pierce the cabbage, and then lift it up over the side. It was easy getting the cabbage off the pitchfork when you rested it on the side of the truck rack. But when the rack was full you had to toss the cabbage into the center of the load.

This was great sport. I was very careful never to lift more than one head at a time while I was pregnant. And if exercise had not been a major part of my life, I would have never succeeded.

If you as a diabetic are not used to exercising, and you want to become active, don't start out like a Babe Zaharias. Take it slow until your body gets used to a certain amount of exercise. Then, if you want more, add a little each day. You will become stronger and you will notice a definite improvement in the way insulin performs in your body. You will almost always need to decrease your insulin or eat more food.

The fall days of late September and early October were beautiful, and cutting cabbage proved a good way to enjoy the outdoors. Often, when I glanced up from my work, a deer would be watching me. As I straightened up to watch the deer, it would skip and run, eventually jumping over a fence at the east end of the field.

This continuous activity made me very cautious of insulin reactions. I never left home without something to eat in my pocket.

The second Sunday in October was our first Wedding Anniversary. Meadville was not the full grown city it is today, and we had a difficult time finding a restaurant to celebrate our special day. We finally located one in Conneaut Lake, enjoying a few hours together. It was a cloudy, grey day, not like the beautiful sunny Saturday when we were married.

In late October the cabbage was finally harvested. Willy hired a man to combine our corn crop. When the first trickle of snow hit the ground, the cattle were all snug in the barn, and we were content, knowing we had more than enough feed to see the animals through the long winter.

Thanksgiving has always been a favorite holiday of mine, but now, as a farmer's wife, the day has taken on special meaning. It usually signifies the end of the outside farm work with crops stored safely for winter's sale or use. We usually welcome the day with a little sigh of relief.

December rolled in, bringing with it some cold, snowy days. On the 16th, after finishing morning chores, Willy and I went to Erie to finish our Christmas shopping. We trudged through the crowds, finally completing everything on our list. It was late when we arrived home, and Willy urged me to stay in the house and rest rather than help with chores. I was tired and gladly took his advice. When my husband finished in the barn, he ate a bite of supper and we went to bed.

Early the next morning I awoke before the alarm sounded with a cramping sensation in my stomach. I called Dr. Ewing. He instructed me to go to the hospital emergency room immediately.

When we arrived, Dr. Ewing examined me and half smiling, said, "I don't think this baby is going to wait until January." He then admitted me to the maternity section of City Hospital and the wait began.

My pains were quite far apart and the doctor urged me to stay very quiet hoping the labor would subside. Everyone was now wondering if the baby was coming ahead of schedule, or if we had simply figured my due date incorrectly.

The afternoon passed quickly, and my labor did not increase. Dr. Ewing did not want me to have this baby naturally because of my problem with insulin reactions, so he scheduled me for a caesarean section the following morning. My husband went home to do chores, after which, a nurse brought me a light supper, along with some medication to relax me. And I slept soundly that night.

The following morning with my labor subsided, a nurse prepared me for surgery. I had never been in an operating room before. I still have my appendix and everyone was now bustling with excitement. Dr. Ewing stopped in. I discovered that he had spent the night at City Hospital, checking me off and on while I slept. I certainly felt fortunate to have an obstetrician like him.

At ten o'clock I was wheeled out in the hall headed for surgery just as my husband came barrelling towards me. The cows, sensing he was pressed for time, refused to cooperate.

Dr. Fred Ewing was also the anesthesiologist, and after being admitted to the brightly lit operating room, he injected a drug into my spinal column, which produced a loss of feeling in the lower part of my body. With the spinal over, I relaxed, and began observing what was taking place.

The surgeon on my right introduced himself, and his assistant, which stood at my left. Several masked nurses were on hand, along with another doctor, and Dr. Gisela Dalrymple, a pediatrician, who was also awaiting the arrival of this baby.

Dr. Ewing stood directly behind me, describing the entire process. I could see the surgeon persistently working, sometimes giving orders to his assistant or the nurses. I was glad I could not see the actual surgery. You know what a coward I am.

After a short time I could tell by their excited tones that they were getting close. I felt a slight twinge when the baby was lifted, and immediately handed to Dr. Dalrymple.

Then, I heard the sound of lusty, robust crying coming from the baby. Dr. Ewing exclaimed, "It is a boy!"

He knew I wasn't a bit surprised.

After that, he said, "Quick, show her." At that point, Dr. Dalrymple walked towards me holding up this beautiful, crying, kicking baby boy.

Dr. Ewing bent down and injected an anesthetic into my intravenous feeding.

"This will put you to sleep while they complete the surgery," he said.

Meanwhile, in all the excitement, everyone had quite forgotten the new father. He kept glancing at his watch realizing that the caesarean must now be history; however, no one looked him up.

He turned the corner where he was pacing back and forth in time to observe a tall, slim figure, dressed in white, place a baby in an isolette behind a glass enclosure. He walked up close, watching intently as she drew a long needle, and properly confiscated blood from the howling infant's foot.

"That must be mine," He mused.

Shortly before they wheeled me down from the recovery room, my husband had finally gotten the word. One week before Christmas, a six-pound, six-ounce, baby boy had been successfully delivered to John and Mary Greene.

How excited we were. Now the strain of previous months dropped from our shoulders.

Dr. Dalrymple wanted to observe the baby in an isolette a few days before issuing him a complete bill of good health. Of course, I more than appreciated the attention she gave him.

According to the nurses, he was a bundle of joy. They pushed my bed down in front of the glass enclosure so I could see him. What a beautiful sight he was.

Naturally, I named him after his father, John W. Greene Jr. John Sr. knew in advance that would happen.

The following day was my husband's birthday. With all the excitement I'd completely forgotten about it. He really wasn't the least bit concerned though, just grateful everything had turned out so well.

We received many cards and letters congratulating us. And Gladys brought me the single rose that had been placed on the pulpit at Bethel Church commemorating John's birth.

A letter arrived from my vivacious, diabetic friend at Bucyrus-Erie expressing her happiness for me. But she also poured out her heart because she was so afraid for herself. She and her boyfriend were now engaged to be married. And her fears of having children were mounting. From my hospital bed I wrote the same account I've written to you, urging her not to be afraid.

A few days after his birth, Dr. Gisela Dalrymple pronounced our baby boy strong and healthy as she placed him in my arms for the very first time. It is truly impossible for me to even try to express what I felt at that moment.

On Christmas day, one week after John's birth, this new mother and father took the tiny baby to his new home. Mother came to help until I got my strength back. And that first Christmas night, while all my house was asleep, I sat by the bassinet tenderly watching the precious figure sleeping so peacefully.

What a wonderful Christmas Day this had been. I was exhausted, but sleep just would not come. As the clock ticked, I reached for my Bible, opening it to the Gospel according to Luke, and began reading:

> And it came to pass in those days, that there went out a decree from Caesar Augustus, that all the world should be taxed.
>
> (And this taxing was first made when Cyrenius was governor of Syria.)
>
> And all went to be taxed, every one into his own City.
>
> And Joseph also went up from Galilee, out of the city of Nazareth, into Judea, unto the

city of David, which is called
Bethlehem; (because he was of
the house and lineage of David;)

To be taxed with Mary his
espoused wife, being great with
child.

And so it was, that, while they
were there, the days were
accomplished that she should be
delivered.

And she brought forth her
firstborn son, and wrapped him
in swaddling clothes, and laid
him in a manger; because there
was no room for them in the inn.

And there were in the same
country shepherds abiding in the
field, keeping watch over their
flock by night.

And, lo the angel of the Lord
came upon them, and the glory
of the Lord shone round about
them; and they were sore afraid.

And the angel said unto them,
fear not; for, behold I bring you
good tidings of great joy, which
shall be to all people.

For unto you is born this day in
the city of David a saviour, which
is Christ the Lord.

And this shall be a sign unto
you; Ye shall find the babe
wrapped in swaddling clothes,
lying in a manger.

And suddenly there was with the

angel a multitude of the
heavenly host praising God, and
saying,
Glory to God in the highest, and
on earth peace, good will toward
men.

Luke 2:1–14.

CHAPTER 9

A Time for Trials

The winter of 1964 assailed us with its blusterly winds. However, I barely noticed the stormy weather for I was busily involved in caring for young John. The incision from my caesarean healed rapidly and I emerged fit as a fiddle. Willy hired a man to help with the farm chores, while I devoted myself entirely to this new profession called motherhood.

The hired man lived with us so I was also responsible for his meals and clean clothes. After a few months, our hired man decided he'd earned enough money and continued on down the road, leaving my husband with a heavy burden of endless chores.

This was a difficult time for me, because I only saw Willy when he took a few minutes off to eat his meals, and then again in the evening when he was totally weary.

Spring came with crops to plant and fences to build. Often, while John was napping, I'd run to the barn, help with a few chores, then back to the house to check on him.

In April of 1964 Dad Kelley passed away. Mother was now in her early sixties, and knowing we would worry about her living alone, Willy and I urged her to come out to the farm and spend the summer with us. She considered the idea and when we disclosed our dire need for an expert babysitter, she consented.

This allowed me some free time to help my husband. It really worked well, because I was never away from John for any extended period of time.

That spring was especially hectic. Besides caring for the cows and planting crops, Willy also spread lime for other farmers. The lime plant was located in Conneaut, Ohio. We live just a few miles from the Ohio border and he hauled lime from the plant, spreading it at the designated farm. I helped in this endeavor by driving a lime spreader to the Conneaut plant, where after it was loaded with the white substance, I would drive it to whatever farm Willy was spreading at.

Bob Thompson finished his freshman year at college and returned to work at our farm, assisting us in whatever activity we were engaged in. Good help is indispensable, especially to farmers. My husband and I felt fortunate we could always count on Bob.

In October of that year, a 110-acre farm located a mile west of our farm was going to be auctioned off. Willy and I were now interested in purchasing additional land to increase the size of our farming operation. We were both looking forward to this auction which would be held the following Saturday. I'd never been to an auction before and I was a bit curious to view this one.

The Friday before the auction my husband and I were busily immersed in evening chores. Willy was milking the cows and I was diligently pushing the grain cart, measuring out the precise amount of grain to each cow.

After completing the east side of the barn, I turned the corner and started up the elevated alleyway towards the cows on the other side. I always tried to gain speed going up this incline so I'd have enough momentum to make it all the way up without stopping. Only a short distance separated me from the landing, when suddenly, a sharp, stabbing pain pierced my right foot!

I let out a shrill scream, pushed the grain cart away, and hobbled helplessly to a bale of straw. Willy heard my cry and ran to help. Holding up my foot, he encountered a small piece of lumber with a nail protruding through it embedded in my foot. He steadied my leg, cautiously pulling the paraphernalia from my foot. The pain was excruciating!

"Can you make it to the house?" He asked. I shook my head "yes."

"Call the emergency room at City Hospital, tell them we'll be there in about forty minutes."

I hobbled to the house, told mother what

had happened, then, went to the telephone where I placed the call to the hospital.

All this time my mind was endeavoring to grasp the seriousness of this situation for a diabetic. Immediately, forboding thoughts of gangrene from a wound that would not heal penetrated my mind. Of all the accidents that could have happened, why did this one have to happen to me?

It was difficult washing and changing clothes, but when my husband finished chores and showered I was ready. While driving to Meadville, we struggled, trying to figure out where that piece of wood came from in the first place. Who was responsible for that protruding nail being in the barn anyway? The answer was beyond both of us.

When we approached City Hospital the pain was unbearable. At this point I really didn't care what they did to my foot. Anything would be better than this.

My doctor met us in the emergency room. Checking my foot, he immediately summoned a surgeon. Meanwhile, a technician appeared, and drew blood from my arm.

"Oh," I groaned, "what a terrible mess I've got myself into now!"

The surgeon walked over and introduced himself.

"I'm Dr. Robert Kirkpatrick." Checking my foot he moaned slightly.

"This is going to hurt, old girl," he quipped, while inserting a local anesthetic into my foot. Then, he administered a tetanus booster.

When my foot was numb, the doctor carefully cleaned the rust and grime from the incision, expounding on why he was using a particular method of treatment. He kept referring to me as "old girl," and I could now smile at his humor because the anesthetic had deadened the pain.

Dr. Kirkpatrick was very curious about my blood glucose level, knowing the danger diabetes presented in this situation. He kept saying to the nurse. "Don't they have that blood sugar done yet?"

The incision was slightly over an inch deep. Willy estimated the nail to have been about two inches long. When the incision was clean, Dr. Kirkpatrick inserted a drain and bandaged my foot. The emergency room nurse walked over to the doctor informing him that my blood glucose was 88.

"Beautiful!" He exclaimed, expressing my thoughts exactly.

"Call my office for an appointment Monday," he instructed, as he handed me some pain pills, "and stay off your foot!"

The ride home was a lot more comfortable, and surprisingly I spent a restful night. The auction was out for me, of course, but when Willy returned home he was grinning.

"It's ours," he said contentedly. I pressed him for details. Only one other person was interested in the property. They stopped bidding after four tries giving my husband a clear shot. He bought the land quite reasonably.

The farm consisted of 110 acres in one continuous piece, and in our part of the country that's a large field. The ground needed quite a bit of clearing. Tile drainage would have to be installed before we could farm it, but it was a start in the right direction.

On Monday afternoon I drove to Dr. Robert

Kirkpatrick's office using my left foot to work the gas pedal. He removed the drain, and checked my foot over carefully. He cautioned me not to put any medication on it.

"This wound must heal from the inside out," he warned. Oh boy, just when I was beginning to think I might beat this thing.

After hearing the doctor's words, those same old worries surfaced. After having diabetes a number of years, would the circulation in my lower legs and feet be good enough to allow this healing? Only time would tell.

Occasionally, I've found myself programmed in such a derogatory manner concerning diabetes that fears of complications can easily overwhelm me. This, of course, was one of those times. I also became engaged in the "why-did-this-have-to-happen-to-me" syndrome, and that kind of thinking can be disastrous.

My attitude definitely needed discipline. Committing this worry to God was absolutely necessary. It's easy for me to believe God's promises when things are going my way, but when things look bleak, it can be a real test of my faith.

The Apostle Paul's life was constantly filled with adversity, yet he never said, "Why did this have to happen to me." In fact, his words reflected quite a different attitude, when, while a prisoner at Rome, he wrote:

> Be anxious for nothing, but in
> everything by prayer and
> supplication with thanksgiving

let your request be known to
God.

And the peace of God, which
surpasses all comprehension,
shall guard your hearts and your
minds in Christ Jesus.

Philippians 4:6,7.

After reading that passage my attitude
disgusted me. When that happened a remarkable
change took place. My thoughts no longer wanted to
dwell on me and my problem, but on how faithful God
has always been to me. How grateful I was for this
instruction.

The following week passed quickly and
each day the pain in my foot lessened. It no longer
hurt when I placed my foot on the floor and I finally
resumed all my old jobs.

Soon, my scheduled appointment with Dr.
Kirkpatrick arrived, and when he checked my foot his
voice boomed, "Beautiful, old girl. Your foot looks just
beautiful! How long have you been a diabetic?" "Seventeen years," I replied.

"That's great," was his response, once
again expressing my thoughts exactly.

Several weeks later he again examined my
foot and afterwards proclaimed my wound to be, "well
healed."

The fall harvest of cabbage and corn progressed smoothly, and December was filled with all
the excitement of Christmas. However, the never ending race to get our farm bookwork caught up to date
always accompanies that month. Farm taxes must be
paid the last day of February, and our farm year ends

December 31, so most farmers look forward to December with the extra burden of making appropriate tax decisions.

The week before Christmas we joyfully celebrated John's first birthday. He is now a grown man, but no December ever passes without our grateful remembrance of his birth.

That winter we bundled our young son up and took him to the barn while we did chores. Sitting in the stroller he'd watch while his dad milked the cows, and his dad in turn kept an eye on him, making sure he stayed in the stroller while I fed the cows and calves.

After our taxes were paid my husband and I drew up a farm budget for the following year. We also did some long range planning as to where we were going and what we wanted to accomplish on the farm. My husband's true love is farming, of course, but raising crops is where that love is strongest. So, our long range plan included purchasing enough farm land which would someday allow us to make our entire living raising farm crops.

Mother spent the winter with Ida and returned the following spring to look after John, who by this time was quite a charge. Somehow he never stayed put for very long.

In the spring of 1965 my brother-in-law, Gerald, purchased his first bulldozer. Consequently, Willy sent him to work clearing 30 acres of the 110-acre farm we recently purchased. And that year a farm drainage contractor installed 13,000 feet of drain tile in the same field.

Our old tractors were not the best and part of our long range plan included replacing them as we became financially able. Shortly before planting time we purchased our first brand new tractor, a 4020 John Deere with an automatic gear shift.

I'm quite sure the John Deere people had city girls turned farm wives in mind when they developed that automatic shift. I loved driving it and spent many hours discing ground just ahead of my husband who was planting crops. We affectionately named that tractor "Jackson." Now we've had our share of bigger and possibly better tractors since then, but after giving us more than 20 years of faithful service, Jackson is still everyone's favorite. That same year we planted most of our farm land to corn, and purchased a new "Gleaner" combine.

My husband continued spreading lime, and in mid July, accepted a contract from the game farm at Cambridge Springs for 125-ton. Willy completed most of the contract and was spreading the next to the last load. I was supposed to drive to the lime plant, get the required tonnage loaded on the truck, then meet my husband at the game farm so he could finish the contract.

It was a beautiful day as I put the truck in gear and pulled away from the scale at the lime plant. However, when I approached the small town of Albion, the truck started making a terrible noise.

It seemed to be coming from the rear of the truck. I looked around, but there didn't seem to be anywhere I could safely pull over. So I continued driving, hoping I could make it into town, but the further I drove the worse the noise got.

It sure would have been nice if I'd taken a mechanic's course sometime in my life. If I'd ever had the slightest idea I would wind up married to a farmer

I certainly would have. I never know what to do if something breaks, so rather than trust my judgment I just kept the noisy truck headed towards the small town.

When I entered the business district people started staring at me and the noisy truck. One man waved his hands frantically, but I just kept on going.

In the center of Albion was a garage. I sighed with relief when I finally pulled the truck to a stop and parked it across the street. While walking towards the garage I glanced back at the truck, and noticed the back wheel on the driver's side was help-lessly tilted.

"How do I get myself into these messes?" I mused, while walking into the garage. I pointed to the truck and said to the owner, "I think I've got a problem."

He doubled over laughing and replied, "Yes, I think you do."

The truck wheel was hanging in such a precarious position that he was afraid he might lose it driving the truck into the garage.

"How much lime do you have on that thing?" He inquired. "Six ton," I replied. He stroked his chin gently, trying to decide what to do about me and that truck.

His helper appeared and the two of them debated on just how to handle the situation. I could not get in touch with my husband, because he was waiting for me in a field at the game farm, and the office on the farm was closed Saturday afternoon. Fi-nally, the men decided, somewhat hesitantly, to drive the truck into the garage. I could then picture my load of lime dumped in the middle of Albion and my husband asking, "What happened?"

I decided I'd tell him I wanted to see the small town GROW, so I contributed his load of lime.

However, they finally did get the truck safely into the garage, and the mechanic explained my problem. Seems like the inner truck wheel was held by a nut and stud. The outer wheel was held by a nut on the inner wheel nut and stud, and the inner wheel nut came loose . . . Understand?

Thank goodness the garage appeared when it did, or the wheel could have fallen off and the truck axle would have been resting on the road.

I'd lost a lot of time, but was grateful everything turned out okay. I did get the load of lime to my husband who was tearing his hair out when I arrived!

It was early afternoon when I started out. With my delay we did not get back home until eight o'clock that evening. The cows were waiting for us at the gate and wobbled uncomfortably into the barn thinking we'd forgotten them.

Nevertheless, that afternoon could have been a disaster for me. As a diabetic I'd already missed a meal, while faced with the responsibility of driving that lime truck safely. A low blood sugar on my part could have spelled danger for others as well as myself.

Many years ago I'd promised myself that I would never drive with a low blood sugar. A small peppermint pattie could never cover for a missed meal, but reaching into my purse I pulled out several neatly wrapped packages of crackers and peanut butter. They were a little stale from being carried around so long, but they were just what I needed.

Driving with a blood sugar below normal can spell trouble for diabetics. That might have been a problem for us in past years, but today, with the inception of the Blood Glucose Monitoring Machine, we have no excuse.

Looking back, that year was also the most significant in terms of farm growth. We were able to borrow enough money allowing us to expand our initial farming operation. We also constructed a farm garage, and purchased several new trucks along with our first grain bin.

Incidentally, when men came to erect the grain bin, John supervised the process. As they hurried along threading bolts into the proper holes, he followed behind removing the bolts. He now accompanied his father everywhere, whether driving truck, milking cows or plowing the back forty. And I began yearning for another baby to complete our family.

The World's Fair was in New York City that year, and in August, the three of us excited about our first vacation headed for the big city. We spent two days at the fair and another day touring the city. It was an active vacation, and I really had to look out for those insulin reactions while walking around the fair. Walking is truly a great exercise for diabetics.

We returned home mentally refreshed. Just getting away from our strenuous schedule a few days revived us. Bob Thompson took good care of the farm work while we were gone, but I'm sure he was glad to relinquish those responsibilities.

In late September, Dr. Fred Ewing confirmed my second pregnancy. My due date was projected around May 1. My control was tight and I was determined to keep it that way to avoid problems with this pregnancy.

Shortly before Thanksgiving a local businessman approached us about buying another farm. The land connected onto the east end of our home farm. My husband told him we were interested, but did not have the money. He, in turn, offered to lend us the money at 3% interest. This was a wonderful opportunity for us, and we knew we'd be foolish to turn it down. However, getting a clear title to the property was a little iffy. It required much time and leg work on the part of that businessman. But we were delighted when he finally succeeded, and we purchased the farm.

That Christmas, Willy's brother and sisters purchased a John Deere pedal tractor for our young son. I never thought two-year olds were capable of career decisions, but little did I realize that as he pumped that tractor around the barn, his future career was already firmly implanted in his mind.

The end of one year and the beginning of the next always brings with it a sense of newness, the chance for a fresh start, and as I eyed the heaping piles of snow from my kitchen window, I wondered just what this year had in store for us.

It seemed a little odd to me, but from the beginning of this pregnancy I sensed a difference from when I carried John. It is not like me to be tired unless my blood sugar is running low. To keep from insulin reactions, I'd tried to keep just a trace of sugar in my urine. So I could not blame this tired feeling on high or low blood sugar levels.

One Sunday afternoon in early February, I again made the foolish mistake of laying down for a short rest after our Sunday dinner. John was napping and my husband was watching a football game on television. Thinking I'd rest for just a half hour I joyfully claimed the living room couch, but to my dismay it turned out to be another fiasco.

I am not a sound sleeper. When John finished napping he tried to wake me. When I did not wake up my husband realized there was trouble. Then, when I did not respond to his treatment of orange juice with sugar, he bundled me up and headed for the emergency room at City Hospital.

My doctor was on vacation at the time and the emergency room nurse summoned a Dr. David Kirkpatrick to my rescue. My husband watched silently as the doctor mixed a medication into a syringe, and inserted the needle directly into the intravenous feeding, which was slowly dripping into my left vein.

"Mary, can you hear me?" The doctor leaned forward trying to command a quick response.

My husband stood with his arms folded and was about to advise this doctor that his wife could not possibly respond in that short a time, but he stepped back, watching in total amazement as I immediately responded to the doctor's question.

"Yes, I can hear you."

Willy was completely dumbfounded! What did Dr. Kirkpatrick use to bring his wife out of that insulin reaction so rapidly? It was nothing less than a miracle according to him.

Dr. Kirkpatrick wanted me to spend the night at the hospital so they could observe me. I'd just begun the last trimester of this pregnancy and keeping those insulin reactions at bay was now a top priority.

Riding home from the hospital the following day, I again listened as my husband described the miraculous treatment Dr. Kirkpatrick used to treat that insulin reaction.

"I really wish you would change doctors," My husband requested.

"Just let me get through this pregnancy," I replied. "I'll think about it then."

"But you really haven't been feeling quite up to par," my husband argued.

"I know, but I'm a little frightened. Just let me get through this pregnancy," I pleaded and our conversation ended.

The month of February slowly drifted past and the winds of March heaped winter's final snow against our white barn. The subject of changing doctors never came up again. I tried to keep my chin up, but I knew something was not right about this pregnancy.

In mid-March, Dr. Ewing advised me to stay off my feet because my legs were slightly swollen. He wanted to see me again in two weeks for another checkup.

During those two weeks my stomach swelled like a balloon. Ann Thompson and I were driving home from the grocery store one afternoon when we were stopped by a policeman conducting a routine traffic check. As he approached my car he was about to ask to see my license, but after looking in the car window, and seeing the size of my stomach he motioned for us to go on. Ann and I had a good laugh about that.

However, on March 29, the day of my scheduled appointment, Dr. Ewing examined me, and even before he spoke I realized something was wrong.

"Your incision is in danger of rupturing, Mary. I want you to go immediately to City Hospital!"

"Just give me one hour," I pleaded.

Reluctantly, he agreed, and I headed towards Springboro to get my husband. Arriving home, I quickly threw some things into an overnight case and together we started for City Hospital.

Dr. Ewing was waiting for us and we could see he was very concerned. He admitted me to the maternity ward and scheduled a caesarean section for eight o'clock the following morning.

Dr. Ewing kept a close watch on me that night. I slept fitfully.

Shortly before eight o'clock the following morning I was wheeled into the operating room. In an effort to save the baby the surgeon made the incision directly over my previous incision.

After a short time I heard a voice exclaim, "Water! It's going everywhere!"

Dr. Ewing moved towards the direction the voice came from, and with all the commotion I could tell there was trouble. After what seemed like an eternity, Dr. Ewing walked towards me and sadly said, "The baby was stillborn."

Waking up in the recovery room, I desperately wanted to believe it had all been a bad dream. The recovery room nurse gently stroked my forehead, assuring me they had done everything they could. I realized that, but I was totally unprepared for the overwhelming sense of loss that encompassed me.

My husband is not a man of endearing words, but when I was finally back in my room, his loving expression only sealed my safekeeping.

"Mary, I married you only because I loved you. We lost this baby, but I don't want to lose you."

He realized the great sense of failure I was experiencing. And his message erased any doubts I might have imagined concerning his support in my now weakened condition.

A nurse entered my room and administered a shot for the pain. Oh, how I wished she could give me a shot to take away the pain that gripped my heart.

In the darkened room I immediately plunged headlong into a deep self-pity, accompanied by the "what-have-I-done-to-deserve-this?" thinking that can easily follow such a calamity.

It seems strange, but another thought quickly permeated my mind, that, of the useless defeat which accompanies this kind of thinking. It was like a tug-of-war was taking place within me, and I began praying:

"Lord, please change my thinking, I feel so helpless, so unable to cope with this loss. Please Lord, take control of this situation." And with that I drifted off to sleep.

Does God really answer prayer? As one that has placed her faith and trust in Him, I can truly answer "yes." However, the answer seldom comes the way we think it should. For when I awoke in that dark, dreary hospital room, Scripture verses I'd learned as a child flooded my heart:

> He is despised and rejected of
> men, a man of sorrows, and
> acquainted with grief; and we
> hid as it were our faces from
> him; he was despised, and we
> esteemed him not.
> Surely he hath borne our griefs,
> and carried our sorrows; yet we
> did esteem him stricken, smitten
> of God and afflicted.
> But he was wounded for our
> transgressions, he was bruised
> for our iniquities; the
> chastisement of our peace was
> upon him; and with his stripes
> we are healed.
> All we like sheep have gone
> astray, we have turned every one
> to his own way; and the Lord
> hath laid on him the iniquity of
> us all.
> He was oppressed, and he was
> afflicted, yet he opened not his
> mouth; he is brought as a lamb
> to the slaughter, and as a sheep
> before his shearers is dumb, so
> he openeth not his mouth.
> He was taken from prison and
> from judgment; and who shall
> declare his generation? For he
> was cut off out of the land of the
> living. For the transgression of
> my people was he stricken.
>
> Isaiah 53:3–8

And Isaiah's prophetic message of Christ's sufferings sunk deep into my being.

There was no instantaneous healing for this loss, only a deep assurance that God does not make mistakes. An all-wise God had given us our firstborn, but chose to take this little boy to be with Himself.

We named him after both grandfathers and laid his tiny body to rest in Spring Cemetery.

The gradual restoration of my strength gave me a renewed challenge to get back home and I was indeed grateful for the young son waiting for me at home.

Within a few days I was discharged from the hospital. Getting back home was indeed wonderful.

However, during a checkup with my doctor the last week of April, my lower legs again appeared swollen. I called this to his attention, but he could not offer me an explanation for this condition. I worked hard keeping my urine sugar in good control, yet continued being tired more often than even I wanted to admit. My incision healed nicely, but the tired feeling would not go away.

"Maybe you need to rest more often," The doctor offered at my next appointment. "Make an appointment to see me in three months."

In the preceding weeks nothing helped this tired, rundown feeling. In fact, rather than improve, it seemed to get much worse and I was constantly dizzy. The dizziness even persisted in bed at night. I no longer had the strength to help outside. Keeping up with the housework along with my young son took every ounce of strength I had.

This was especially frustrating, because my diabetes was in excellent control. My urine tests revealed little sugar before meals or at bedtime.

My husband was becoming increasingly concerned about my condition and urged me to return to the doctor for another checkup.

It was the middle of May when I again sat facing the doctor, who by this time was completely baffled with my condition.

"Come see me again in a month," He exclaimed, after examining me. "If you're not any better I'll have to admit you to the hospital and run some tests."

Willy was disgusted when I relayed the doctor's words to him. I also wondered how I would ever make it another month.

Two weeks later I walked outside to give our dog Lady some leftovers, but when I started back towards the house I staggered from the dizziness.

"I'll never make it back," I gasped, "If only I had something to hold onto."

Unbeknown to me, my husband was watching from the feed room door. Now with his patience sorely tried, he picked up the barn telephone and immediately phoned the doctor.

"If you don't do something for Mary, she's not going to make it!" he said with despair.

"Take her to City Hospital, I'll meet you there," The doctor replied.

"Pack whatever you'll need," Willy spoke gently as he approached me from behind. Taking my arm to steady me, he continued, "We're going to the hospital."

This time I was glad to be headed for the hospital, because without a doubt, something was certainly wrong with me.

After being admitted, I willingly collapsed into the clean hospital bed while my thoughts paralleled Willy's. Perhaps I wouldn't make it this time.

Soon, a slim young lady from the lab drew two large vials of blood from my arm. Later that afternoon, the head nurse appeared with what I thought was an intravenous feeding. Yet, when I looked closer, it was not an intravenous, but a blood transfusion.

When I questioned the nurse, she replied, "You are severely anemic. We will be doing tests to determine what is causing it."

"Anemic!" That really shocked me. I never dreamed I'd be diagnosed anemic. I've always been strong and healthy. Why that's a term I'd always associated with weak, deficient people, not me! Nevertheless, it was me. This once, healthy diabetic woman was now anemic.

After finding a vein, the nurse inserted the needle. I slept off and on while the blood dripped slowly into my vein. Several hours later the pouch was empty and a nurse removed the needle from my arm.

The following morning I was amazed at how good I felt, practically like my old self. Did that blood transfusion do that?

I then recalled a verse of Scripture which says:

> For the life of all flesh is its blood.
>
> Leviticus 17:14

I'd certainly found that to be true. What a difference the blood transfusion made. I tossed back the sheet, and was about to hop out of bed when a nurse pushing a cart entered my room.

"Ah-ah-ah, get back in bed," She jested. "I've got to run some tests on you."

Reluctantly, I swung my feet back onto the bed.

"What kind of tests?" I asked. She mumbled the word leukemia half under her breath, and as I continued questioning her, she mentioned that they were also looking for "possible internal bleeding."

Her words did not frighten me. They only sparked an intense desire to know what was causing this anemia.

Later that afternoon I sat in the hospital lounge waiting for my mother-in-law, who was bringing John to see me. When they entered the lounge he romped towards me . . . Now, almost three, he was certainly the picture of health. Crawling up on my lap we talked about the farm and how he was helping his dad with all the work. When visiting hours were over, I watched sadly as they walked down the hospital corridor and out the door.

Remaining in the lounge, I began talking with another patient when a nurse entered. "Mrs. Greene?" She looked at both of us, not quite sure which one was Mrs. Greene. As I nodded my head in response, she said, "They want to run another test on you now."

Returning to the room, I thought about my visit with John while a technician drew more blood from my vein.

Later that evening, after visiting hours were over, my husband slipped in. If I thought I had troubles what a strain this illness was on him. It was now the beginning of June, he was trying to keep the farm running smoothly, with a young son to care for, while his wife was confined to a hospital with some kind of mystifying illness. However, we both tried to keep our spirits up, especially in front of each other hoping they would soon find the answer.

The next few days hummed with activity as more tests were taken. Each day I questioned my doctor as to what the tests revealed and each day I got the same answer, "Nothing."

The days drifted into weeks. I tried to content myself with hospital living, but much to my dismay I soon slipped back into the same weakened condition. I watched quietly as the nurse probed my arm, looking again for a good vein to transfuse blood. When all was still, I watched the blood dripping slowly from the elevated container through the sterile tube and into my vein.

These were frustrating days, not only for my family and me, but for the doctor as well. He had literally exhausted all resources in his search for the cause of this anemia.

In August he released me from the hospital, but only to see me return in the same weakened condition. The days passed slowly with little assurance I'd ever recover.

I was permitted to spend Labor Day weekend at home. To celebrate the holiday my mother-in-law hosted a picnic, inviting Ann McLallen and her parents. It was a beautiful day and I was happy to be with my family and friends. I tried hard to forget my troubles, but before my friend left she squeezed my hand saying, "Mary, I'm so concerned."

How well I understood her feelings. There just didn't seem to be any hope for me.

Returning to the hospital, my doctor mentioned that he would be on vacation a few days. Another doctor would be caring for me along with his other patients.

The next morning Dr. David Kirkpatrick walked into my hospital room holding my chart in his hand. This was the same Dr. Kirkpatrick that brought me out of the insulin reaction so rapidly. He is also a brother to Dr. Robert Kirkpatrick, the surgeon who took care of my foot injury. Dr. Kirkpatrick asked me a few questions and told me he had been studying my chart.

"I've ordered a test which will be done tomorrow morning," He said, sounding hopeful. However, I really didn't have much hope. After all this time, I was afraid it would only mean another disappointment.

The following morning a nurse and technician walked into my room.

"This will be a little uncomfortable," the technician said. He held up a long rubber tube. "We want you to keep swallowing while we work this tube down your throat."

At first I thought I'd gag, but they urged me to relax and keep swallowing, while they worked precisely with the tube. Soon, the young man held up his hand and I stopped swallowing. A few minutes later he pulled the tube out and the test was completed.

The test is known as a Gastric Analysis. I wondered what a test like that could reveal.

The following morning, Dr. Kirkpatrick entered my room with a smile on his face. The test had indeed proven successful. It revealed a vitamin deficiency.

Red blood cell production takes place in the bone marrow, and depends substantially on two vitamins, vitamin B12, and folic acid. Our body absorbs these vitamins from certain foods. If we do not get enough of either vitamin, red blood cell production fails. Also, those red blood cells that are formed are defective. The result is either a B12 deficiency or a folic acid deficiency.

In a healthy person the liver contains reserves of vitamin B12. If you develop an inability to absorb vitamin B12, your body will eventually deplete these reserves and anemia will develop.

Our bodies normally absorb vitamin B12 from the lower small intestine. Before this can occur the vitamin must combine in the stomach with a special substance known as intrinsic factor, which is secreted by the stomach lining. In some people, for reasons that are not fully understood, the stomach lining stops secreting enough intrinsic factor. Without it, sufficient quantities of vitamin B12 cannot be absorbed.

Once our ability to absorb vitamin B12 through the digestive tract has been lost, it can never be regained. But the treatment for this deficiency was simple: an injection of vitamin B12, once or twice a week.

The treatment sounded so simple, so reasonable, I almost had trouble believing it. Thoughts of another injection didn't phase me at all. In fact, it really seemed too good to be true.

A nurse instructed me with my first injection of the vitamin. The following day I was released from the hospital.

I wasted little time calling Dr. David Kirkpatrick's office for a future appointment. However, he was so busy I had to wait eight months for that appointment. But I was now convinced he was a doctor well worth waiting for.

All of us would rather enjoy life's blessings than face its trials, yet both are part of our lives. But as this poem says:

> Looking back, it seems to me
> all the grief, which had to be,
> left me when the pain was o're
> richer than I'd been before.
>
> —Anon

After my long summer confined at City Hospital, I certainly found that to be true.

Getting back home to my family and being able to enjoy good health again seemed like a miracle to me. I don't take good health for granted anymore. It is a very special gift, one I will always be grateful for.

My husband had done an excellent job during my long absence, and once again, I was reminded of the loving, caring family God has blessed me with.

That fall we purchased our second grain bin for the farm, and when our cabbage was ready to harvest, I plunged into the work with a new enthusiasm delighted, once again, to be able to help with the farm chores along with caring for my home and family.

My first appointment with Dr. David Kirkpatrick occurred in April of 1967. After years of numerous doctor's examinations, I must admit, that when Dr. Kirkpatrick completed the checkup, I really felt confident. I would soon be classed as a long-term diabetic. During my appointment, the doctor thoroughly examined my eyes, tested my reflexes, and carefully checked my feet for a pulse.

He suggested an insulin change from NPH to a combination of Semilente and Ultralente insulins, 20 units of each for a total of 40 units. And I accomplished that change myself without being admitted to a hospital.

Why did he allow me to tackle the change myself? After many years of good control, he knew he could trust my judgment in this matter, and if I had any problem, he was only a phone call away.

I really appreciated his confidence, because, when we enter a hospital for insulin changes we can't always get a true picture of our control, especially, if we are active.

Many people live with the impression that all diabetics have to do is watch what they eat. However, you and I know this is completely false! We must carefully watch three different details that are all a part of the complete structure of control: insulin, exercise, and eating. The proper blending of these three allows for a perfect balance, but it isn't always easy.

Let me give you an example: A woman I knew was diagnosed with diabetes and required insulin. After her release from the hospital, she experienced her first reaction to that insulin while home alone one day. Her husband found her staggering around the house when he returned from his golf game.

She had been warned about insulin reactions while still in the hospital, but she was totally unprepared when it happened. In fact, afterwards, she experienced a deep depression that lasted for days.

After talking with her, I was most grateful that I had experienced insulin reactions while still in the hospital. How helpful it would have been if she could have also experienced her first insulin reaction while still under the proper supervision.

Some diabetics have a keen sense of low blood glucose levels, but others are not as fortunate. This situation might have been avoided if her doctor had prescribed a few extra units of insulin, allowing her to experience an insulin reaction while still in the hospital. She could have been checked closely during that time, and if she had trouble diagnosing the insulin reaction herself, then I would suggest starting all over again until she learned to recognize them.

Sometimes we can determine the cause of insulin reactions, and sometimes we can't. But my friend decided to clean her house that day. That was something she had done often prior to the discovery of her diabetes; however, after that discovery and control with insulin, she was functioning under different circumstances.

If insulin reactions are going to be a part of our lives, and I'm convinced they will be when we try to maintain good control, then we should be prepared to handle those reactions properly.

November 4, 1967, was supposed to be

D-Day for me. It had now been 20 years since my diabetes was diagnosed.

Please don't be frightened by these 20-year tales. I always listened in horror to them myself, until I finally realized that the only stories told about diabetics today are the sad ones. They've taken their toll. People are indeed terrified of this "problem." In fact, when I mentioned that I was writing about my life as a diabetic to one man in the medical field, he said:

"You'd better not, something bad might happen!" It was easy to see he still insisted on living in the dark ages concerning diabetic management.

Don't get me wrong. I'm not making light of diabetic complications. They can happen. In fact, during my first few years with this "problem," thanks to Miss X, I was sure each new year was going to be my last until I finally learned to relax with this "problem," controlling my diabetes one day at a time, forgetting about tomorrow.

Consequently, I discovered as shall you, that with good control complications will have a difficult time squeezing into our lives.

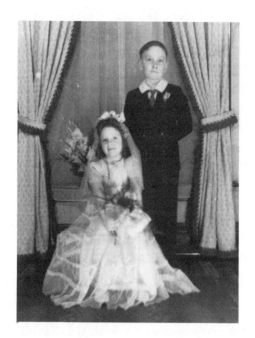

Mary & Bill in Gladys & Wally's wedding—1943

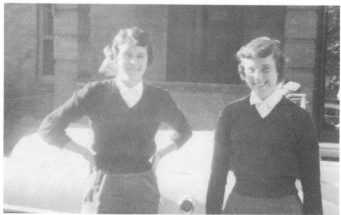

Cynthia left, and Mary standing beside yellow convertible—1955

The Family
1970

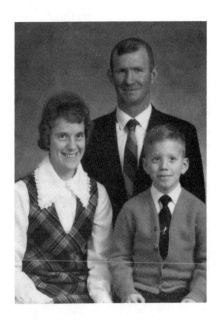

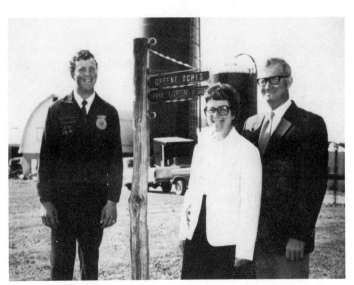

Picture taken for John's Eastern Region Future Farmers of America competition—1985

CHAPTER 10

More Ups Than Downs

During the spring of 1968 we planted over 400 acres of field corn and enough oats to use in our dairy operation. After the first crop hay was in the barn, we also planted 12 acres of kraut cabbage.

In October, we purchased another 100 acres of ground which connected onto the east end of our farm. 27 acres of that ground was well-drained, creekbottom land, but the remaining acres required tile drainage.

That fall we cut and delivered cabbage to the Albro Packing Company in between caring for the cows morning and evening. At night my husband shelled corn.

After filling several trucks with the wet

grain he would come home. We'd wake John, bundle him up, and off we would go, each driving a loaded truck to Conneautville, a small town only a few miles away, where men unloaded the corn into a small grain dryer at the Conneautville Farmers Exchange.

Mr. David Johns owned this feed mill. My husband, young John, and myself, had a true friend in Mr. Johns.

While we waited, Mr. Johns would always treat John to a cup of hot cocoa in his office. If he thought we were wretched parents for getting that little boy up each night he never said, but one thing I do know, our young son was always ready to go to Mr. Johns' feed mill day or night.

Thinking back today, it's hard to believe we ever survived those hectic years. But strong in our favor was our unprecedented desire to succeed in the occupation we loved.

After our cabbage harvest was completed, my husband concentrated his efforts on shelling corn. One morning following our barn ritual, I suggested he stay with the corn harvest rather than losing the time it took to do evening chores. He looked at me kind of funny, and said, "Do you mean you want to milk them yourself?"

"Sure!" I replied.

I'd been helping milk the last few cows each morning after the feeding was finished, so why not do it all. I really didn't know how he could keep up the pace he'd set for himself anyway. And this would just speed up our harvest a bit.

He gave me his famous grin while issuing specific instructions on certain cows. That evening I performed my first solo with those Holstein cows.

Cows are a lot like people. Each one is just a little different. Some are loving and lick each other while waiting to be milked and others, well, you'd better approach them cautiously if you don't want to get a swift kick! Knowing this, I worked warily the first few evenings, allowing the cows and me time to get used to each other.

When I first began taking 40 units of the combined insulins my activities did not include milking 42 cows. I was feeding cows morning and evening, along with driving tractor for spring planting. But when our cabbage harvest started, and I was emerged in physical activity all day long, that 40 units of insulin was way too much. Had I continued taking that dosage, I probably would have been mistaken for a cabbage head sprawled in the field.

However, when I started adjusting my insulin to these activities, I thought I would only need to cut down on the Semilente insulin which has a 2–8 hour peak, but I was wrong. The benefits of exercise are so tremendous to diabetics.

Nevertheless, that first self-adjustment of a new insulin was a real burden to my husband. Many mornings he cradled my head in his left arm, while spooning orange juice with sugar down my throat with his right hand. What a way . . . to start your day!

If only I had consulted Dr. Kirkpatrick I could have saved my husband that unpleasant task. I soon realized that the extended benefits of my activities also required a cut in the Ultralente insulin. And while I was engaged in that strenuous work my entire insulin dosage was reduced by 15 units.

It requires a sustained effort to correctly

reduce our insulin before exercising, but as far as I'm concerned the benefits far outweigh the trouble.

My next scheduled appointment with Dr. Kirkpatrick was during this busy season. After my examination we discussed the problems associated with reducing insulin when necessary, along with my problem prior to the correct insulin reduction. Before I left his office he gave me a prescription for Glucagon, which could be used in extreme emergencies to treat a severe insulin reaction.

Glucagon is a naturally occurring substance produced by the pancreas. It is advantageous because it enables the patient to produce his own blood sugar to correct the hypoglycemic state until the patient can take carbohydrates by mouth. It comes in two separate vials, which must be mixed properly in a syringe, and injected into the patient the same as insulin.

What a blessing Glucagon is to family members treating a diabetic in severe insulin shock. Just knowing it's available gives substantial security to them as well as us. However, having that medication is no excuse for poor control on our part.

Low blood sugars will be a normal part of our diabetic walk when we try to maintain good control, but severe insulin shock, occurring regularly, definitely calls for more prudent behavior on the part of the diabetic. Glucagon has been in our house some 19 years now, and only used once.

During the next several years our farming operation progressed rapidly. We added two new John Deere tractors to our fleet, a third grain bin, and another 100 acres of well-drained ground to our farm.

Mother was now spending a few months each summer with us and the balance of the summer with Ida and her family. She secured a small apartment in Miami, Florida, where she lived during our long, cold Pennsylvania winters.

In September of 1969, I watched apprehensively as a curly headed lad climbed onto the school bus for the first time. His father and I labored to prepare him for this event. But I had quite forgotten to prepare myself. I spent a fretful afternoon, all to no avail. A few hours later, he hopped off the school bus grinning from ear to ear. His first day at kindergarten had gone amazingly well and he adjusted beautifully to this new undertaking.

During the spring of 1970 we planted four acres of strawberries, which would not be ready for harvest until the following year. The strawberries were planted as a specialty crop for us, and in reality, fulfilled a lifelong dream for my husband, who always longed to raise this bright delicious fruit.

One afternoon Mr. Johns stopped. As he and I sat on the porch steps, he began talking, "Mary, I want you to do something for me."

I gave him my full attention. "I want you to talk John (remember, only the family calls him Willy) into serving on the school board. We had a resignation at our meeting last night and I think John would be perfect for the job."

We live in what is known as the Conneaut Valley area of Crawford County, which is comprised of two very small towns, of which each had separate schools with grades one thru twelve, and three townships who each had elementary schools. Many years before the word merge was even popular, this community had the foresight to build a modern high school, and a separate grade school for the entire area.

With this sometimes difficult transition completed in our district, I was quite sure my husband would enjoy the challenge of serving on the board, but where would he ever get the time?

Later that evening I relayed Mr. Johns request to Willy and we discussed the pros and cons. He realized that accepting it would require a sacrifice for him, as well as our farm. However, living in a country with the freedom to pursue his dream, had also produced in him a sense of responsibility towards that country, and he accepted.

Mr. Johns was elated with his decision. And his appointment was unanimously approved at the next school board meeting.

During the years my husband and I had worked prudently, carefully managing our spending to keep our indebtedness intact. Consequently, on a warm August morning in 1970, I drove to the Conneautville Bank with a check tucked inside my purse written in the full amount of our mortgage.

When the young woman behind the window exclaimed, "You want to pay this off!" I thought I was going to lose it as I fought back tears of joy. Then, I suddenly regained my composure, and with a generous smile stepped forward, remarking, "I sure do." With such confidence, it even startled me.

Knowing that everything belonged to us, rather than us and the bank was indeed a great accomplishment. But this was not the time to stop and pat ourselves on the back. We still had a long way to go.

My husband and I have plenty of faults,

but pride is not one of them. Nothing could have humbled us more.

The following morning while reading in the Psalms, one verse in particular multiplied that feeling.

> The Lord is my strength and my
> shield, my heart trusted in him,
> and I am helped, therefore my
> heart greatly rejoiceth, and with
> my song will I praise him.
>
> Psalm 28:7

Cabbage harvest would soon be in full swing, and so one Friday morning in mid-September I tackled the fall house cleaning with a vengeance. I labored relentlessly, tackling one job after the other.

I'd cut my insulin a few units that morning knowing I was going to clean, but the way I was going at it a few units was not enough. I finished a kitchen window just as John hopped off the school bus. He walked in the door, threw his reading book on the kitchen table, and announced; "Mom, your sugar is low!"

Well, of all the audacity! Who did that little first grader think he was anyway telling me my sugar was low. My first reaction was to bop him one, but not being a violent woman, I plopped down on a kitchen chair, arguing with him while he got the orange juice out of the refrigerator, stirred a spoonful of sugar into it, and insisted that I drink it.

Oh, why do those low blood sugars make us so irritable and argumentive? I realized my blood sugar was low before I started cleaning that last window, and fully intended to eat something the minute the window was finished.

That situation would have never occurred had I eaten something the minute I suspected a low blood sugar.

You and I must be especially careful to avoid problems like this. That little boy's feelings were really hurt and by the one person who would have protected and defended him against any enemy. Now, I was the enemy. I can still hear his voice pleading with me, "Mom, please drink it!"

It was the sound of his pitiful, young voice that finally persuaded me to pick up the glass and drink the juice. In a few minutes I was my old self again, but I'd shattered the feelings of my young son.

This is a touchy problem which some diabetics choose to ignore; however, we really can't afford to ignore it. Later that evening Willy and I spent time with John, discussing the trauma this episode surely caused him.

He, of course, had done the right thing. I was the guilty party. If you've experienced the same problem, discussing it with your family is a must. Be sure to let them know how much you appreciate their help in situations like this.

But don't forget how extremely difficult it is for the person trying to help a diabetic who absolutely refuses help. Just put yourself in their shoes for a change. If hurt feelings become a real problem, try and work out an agreement for future insulin reactions.

As a diabetic, I can honestly tell you that I had to work on myself. Apparently, we reach a point in our hypoglycemic state where we just will not listen.

Nevertheless, you can program yourself to cooperate even when you don't want to. It might sound absurd, but I know it's true because I do it. Whenever my husband or son says, "Your sugar is low." That immediately initiates two responses: First, keep my mouth shut!, Second, drop whatever I'm doing and eat something quickly.

In previous years diabetics didn't have much hope for that problem, but today with the proper use of the Blood Glucose Monitoring Machine, we can diagnose those low blood sugar levels before they become a real problem.

On the other hand, please remember, dear family, that all diabetics long for perfect control. That might be possible, if we continually sat or reclined, had balanced meals served to us, and did not lift a finger, other than to inject ourselves with the proper amount of insulin. But what kind of life would that be?

I know I've spent a lot of time talking about low blood sugars, probably, because they have been my number one problem. But if the diabetic man or woman in your life is practicing good control while maintaining an active lifestyle, don't throw in the towel because of a few insulin reactions. However, if they are occurring too frequently, then your diabetic definitely needs their physician's help. Otherwise, start encouraging them in the proper use of the Blood Glucose Monitoring Machine to help avoid these situations.

That fall during my regular examination, Dr. Kirkpatrick discovered a cataract in my right eye.

Cataracts are fairly common among older adults and long term diabetics are especially prone to them.

"Don't worry about it," was my doctor's good advice. "It will be many years before you will need anything done." He was absolutely right.

Combining my active life as a farmer's wife with my "problem" of diabetes hasn't always been easy, but it has been rewarding. In the spring of 1971 we anxiously anticipated our first strawberry crop. While the large green berries turned red, I walked the rows with a small spade shovel removing stray weeds from the lush foliage.

At last the crop was ready, so we advertised our first "pick your own." We soon discovered people love this fruit and we realized that strawberries were going to play a significant part in our farming operation.

That year we also purchased a grain dryer. Having a dryer would eliminate those countless trips to the feed mill hauling wet grain. It would certainly simplify our grain drying operation.

Willy enjoyed the challenge the school board presented, but that July our district was given a state mandate to merge with the Linesville and Conneaut Lake districts, making one district which covered a total area of 318 square miles.

At a special May meeting three men were going to be elected from the previous seven man board to serve on the newly merged school board. Much to my husband's surprise, he was one of the men chosen.

That fall, our long exhausting days of corn and cabbage harvest progressed rapidly. When I finished the evening chores I was weary. At that time we

135

had 42 stanchions in our barn, 21 on a side, each filled with Holstein cows. Now I had plenty of energy when I started milking each evening, but after a hard day, I was really tired when I got up to the walkway, and I had fourteen more cows to milk above the walkway.

One morning while doing chores together, I said to my husband, "Why don't we sell those fourteen cows above the walk? It would really make things a lot easier."

Of course, he realized I was tired at the end of a demanding day. So he put his arm around me and ever so tenderly explained, "Honey, the milk we produce up to the walkway just pays the bills, but the milk we produce from the 14 cows above the walk is our profit."

Why did I share that experience with you? Because it changed my attitude. Consequently, when I milked those fourteen cows above the walk each evening I could whistle, because the bills were paid, and now it was pure profit.

Attitude! It affects all of us. And your attitude in relation to your diabetes can spell success or failure in your diabetic walk. Don't allow this "problem" to drag you down, it can become a valuable asset if only you will let it.

In October, we introduced Ann McLallen to a handsome neighbor, Carl Pepper. When Ann and her family joined us for Thanksgiving dinner that year I sensed a touch of romance in the air.

This was an excellent time to be grain farming. Our markets were strong and the opportunities seemed endless. In late December we decided it was time to reduce some of our work load, and in keeping with our original plan, we put our Holstein cows up for sale.

It seems rather ironic, but we did not have an auction. In fact, we never advertised them. The word got out that they were for sale. And one evening in January of 1972, a man walked into our barn, looked at the cows and bought them immediately.

We kept the heifers and calves, but with the milk cows gone it was like being on vacation. However, we soon discovered that we are creatures of habit. The alarm no longer rang at 5:30 each morning, but would you believe my husband and I would both be wide awake at that unfriendly hour.

Habits are hard to break. That's why it's so important for us to establish good habits in regard to our diabetes. And it's never too late to start. If you've been lax in your control, I hope you'll begin again to renew those good habits. You won't be sorry you did.

That December my husband was elected to a 6-year term on the Conneaut School Board, realizing that somehow he would find the time for that important job.

In February of 1972, we placed an order with our local John Deere dealer for a 7520 tractor. This tractor is a four-wheel drive with duals on each drive, and a draw-bar horsepower of 175. In March we traveled to the John Deere tractor works in Waterloo, Iowa, where we were given the opportunity to watch a 7520 tractor assembled.

Honestly, I could not believe the size of that tractor, it looked like a monster to me. John was feasting his eyes on it with an expression only an eight year old boy is capable of. At the end of the assembly line, when they let him climb up in the cab of that tractor, he looked like he'd been to heaven and back.

We proceeded to tour the plant while a guide explained each operation. Towards the end of the tour our guide paused behind a middle-aged man busily engaged in his work. Before the guide uttered a word I realized the man was blind.

Our guide spoke to him, and he smiled at us. When we were several yards away, the guide informed us that the man had worked at the John Deere plant some twenty-two years, and was blinded in an automobile accident outside the plant. However, he continued working, and had a very positive outlook on life.

You will never know what meeting that blind man did for me.

That evening, while reading the menu in a Waterloo restaurant, my thoughts returned to the blind man, who refused to let himself become a burden to society because he was disabled.

From Waterloo, we drove to the John Deere International Headquarters in Moline, Illinois, where they treated us to an elegant lunch, along with a tour of the combine and plow works. But somehow I just could not stop thinking about the blind man. Attitude! Without uttering a word that man's life said it all.

Diabetes certainly hasn't dulled my senses for in April of that year, Willy and I were the attendants at the wedding of our friends Ann McLallen and Carl Pepper. They had a lovely dinner after the evening ceremony. I ate prior to the occasion, eliminating any danger of an insulin reaction.

That spring, I pulled a disc behind our new 7520 tractor. Driving it was pure luxury. Sitting in the air-conditioned cab I was protected from the hot sun. When I climbed out of the cab after dark, I was clean! What a difference. Usually, on an ordinary tractor my eyes would be filled with dirt and my skin covered with dust. We named that work horse, Paul Bunyan, after the giant lumberjack, who in American folk-lore performed superhuman feats.

One Friday afternoon shortly after strawberry harvest, I went to Dr. Kirkpatrick's office for my scheduled appointment. During the examination he discovered a lump in my left breast. He was quite concerned. That same afternoon he arranged for me to be examined by a surgeon after which the surgeon scheduled my admittance to City Hospital Sunday afternoon with surgery to take place Monday morning.

What a frightening experience: one tiny lump which could indicate the presence of cancer. But right now worry was the worst thing I could do. Those anxious, troubled feelings, coupled with my imagination, would only frustrate me. I could not allow that to happen.

But isn't this what life is all about anyway: a mixture of joy, sorrow, happiness, and trials? On my drive home that afternoon, I began considering the various joys and trials of my life until now. And much to my delight the joys far outweighed the trials.

That evening I focused my thoughts on a much loved Psalm, written some 3000 years ago. We often hear this Psalm quoted at funerals, and while it offers comfort in death, it also offers strength for the living.

The Lord is my Shepherd; I shall
not want.

He maketh me to lie down in
green pastures; he leadeth me
beside the still waters.

He restoreth my soul; he leadeth
me in the paths of righteousness
for his name's sake.

Yea, though I walk through the
valley of the shadow of death, I
will fear no evil; For thou art
with me; Thy rod and thy staff
they comfort me.

Thou preparest a table before me
in the presence of mine enemies;
thou anointest my head with oil;
my cup runneth over.

Surely goodness and mercy shall
follow me all the days of my life,
and I will dwell in the house of
the Lord forever.

Psalm 23.

After reading that Psalm, I could then picture a shepherd caring for his helpless sheep on rough
and rocky terrains. And I knew I could trust the Good
Shepherd to see me through this uncertain time.

That Sunday, following our morning
church service we went out to dinner. I didn't have a
Blood Glucose Monitoring Machine back then, but I
knew from testing my urine each day, precisely what
my blood glucose level would be by the time I reached
the hospital.

Did you ever check your blood glucose level to see how long it takes before your blood glucose returns to normal after eating a meal? If not, try it. Knowing that can really help in maintaining good control.

When my lab work was completed, I returned to the office at City Hospital and signed my name to a consent form, which would allow the surgeon to remove my breast if it was cancerous. Nevertheless, through the entire ordeal I maintained a deep peace.

After being admitted, I was disappointed to find the other bed in my room empty. When my family went home I began reading a book I'd stuck in my overnight case. However, when a nurse came to take my temperature and pulse I was sure I had some communicable disease. It was almost like she was afraid to touch me.

I'm not at all sure what that book was about, but it must have been interesting because I finished it that night. The following morning a nurse tried to be pleasant as she prepared me for surgery. But honestly, I felt like I had bad breath.

Soon, a technician started an intravenous feeding, and before long, I slowly edged from my bed onto the waiting surgical cart.

The operating room was freezing cold. A kind nurse brought extra blankets to cover me. The last thing I remember was watching the anesthesiologist inject an anesthetic into my intravenous feeding.

When I awoke in the recovery room I was warm as toast. I remember thinking how good it felt to be warm. Before I had time to reflect on anything else, a nurse bent over me, and with a broad, beaming smile announced, "It was benign."

Back in my room I felt like a celebrity when nurses I'd never seen before dashed in and out of my room chatting happily. It was then I realized what a fragile, fearful world I had entered for just a little while.

CHAPTER 11

A Change of Pace

In January of 1973 my family and I boarded a 737 airplane at Chicago's O'Hara Field bound for Dallas, Texas. This was the first time John or I had ever flown on a commercial airplane. I must admit I was really impressed. Our flight was smooth. I could hardly contain my excitement because our final destination was Honolulu, Hawaii.

At Dallas we boarded a Braniff 747 for our flight over the Pacific Ocean to the island of Oahu. We were among the last group boarding the plane. To my dismay we could not find three seats together. The stewardess finally located two separate end seats for John and myself. A pleasant middle-aged couple urged John to sit beside them in the seat directly behind me near the front of the plane, while my husband took the very last of four seats along the back wall of the gigantic airplane.

We barely had enough time to fasten our seat belts before the plane was in the air. All I could do was gaze in amazement at the size of it.

When the announcement was made allowing us to unfasten our seat belts, the young man sitting behind me tapped me on the shoulder saying, "This is the only way to go mom."

A farm magazine we subscribed to had been featuring Hawaiian vacations. In November of the previous year we decided to spend a week on the islands with this tour group.

That was before diabetic publications featured articles on travel for diabetics, and knowing MYSELF well kept me out of a lot of trouble.

The morning we boarded the airplane, I cut both the Semilente and Ultralente insulins a few units to avoid possible insulin reactions. It's a good thing I did, because our flight across the ocean was rough, due to a very large storm system over the Pacific.

My prime reason for cutting the insulin, however, was knowing how excited I would be. Excitement always lowers my blood glucose level. Let's face it, how could anyone take their first major airplane flight without getting excited!

Nevertheless, halfway through the flight my excitement waned. As I watched one stewardess after the other race up and down the aisle gathering those little bags passengers had put to good use. If I were a young woman, this glamorous occupation as an airline stewardess would have suddenly lost its allure.

A voice over the loudspeaker requested we fasten our seat belts. While turbulence buffeted the gigantic airplane, the young man behind me slept peacefully.

As the airplane made its landing approach, the stewardess insisted on waking him. I'm sure I don't have to tell you what happened after that.

However, all was forgotten when we stepped into the airport at Honolulu and lovely Hawaiian maidens slipped beautiful leis around our neck. The fresh flowers were exquisite. What a wonderful welcome to an enchanting island.

As we walked into the open lobby at the Sheraton Waikiki, the ocean breezes stirred the wind chimes. What a beautiful sound.

The view from our room was lovely. After freshening up, we took a short rest to relax our still weaving heads. We all need time away from our daily routine. Vacations are as essential to diabetics as they are to everyone else. However, we can't afford to neglect our diabetic management routine which will allow us the vitality to enjoy our vacations.

If we weren't touring we were shopping. How could anyone not help loving these beautiful islands with their graceful palm trees.

After flying to the island of Kauai, we reveled in the beauty of the Fern Grotto, a hidden cave framed by giant ferns with an 80-foot waterfall, plunging from above the grotto to the rocks below. People travel from around the globe to get married at that romantic spot.

We stopped to view the Waimea Canyon, a beautiful, colored gorge 2000 feet deep. We also dropped by a pineapple farm to learn how they grow this juicy tropical fruit.

Of course, all good things must come to an end, and after visiting many places of interest, it was soon time to leave. We were grateful our flight home was relatively smooth. This time we sat together while John chatted about our tour of Pearl Harbor, which was the highlight of our vacation for him.

In mid-February I attended a 2-day Fruit and Vegetable Grower's Seminar conducted by the Pennsylvania State University at State College, Pennsylvania. We were very new in the strawberry business. At that seminar I learned much about growing and marketing that crop.

When traveling alone I always wear my "I am a diabetic" necklace. I must admit, I really hated wearing it when I was young, thinking the card in my wallet was enough. However, maturity helped me realize that this necklace is also important, especially when traveling alone.

At my spring appointment Dr. Kirkpatrick introduced me to Dr. John Nesbitt, a young doctor who had completed his residency in the practice of internal medicine. Dr. Nesbitt would now be practicing medicine in the same office with Dr. David Kirkpatrick.

In an effort to lighten Dr. Kirkpatrick's work load, some of his patients were going to be turned over to Dr. Nesbitt. I would be seeing Dr. John Nesbitt at my next appointment. This was not a permanent arrangement, only a temporary one. At a future time I would be transferred back to Dr. Kirkpatrick.

That spring, along with our other crops,

we planted over 100 acres of oats to sell on the open market. A carpenter friend also built us a roadside stand from which to sell picked strawberries. After painting the stand inside and out, I painted several huge red strawberries on the pure white stand, along with our farm name, which I painted in green after the luscious, looking strawberries.

Willy organized a crew to help him with the pick-your-own operation. After purchasing white short sleeve shirts for each crew member, I sewed a large red strawberry on the back so customers could easily recognize the people in charge.

While the pick-your-own activity bustled, I was in charge of a separate crew, responsible for keeping that neat, looking strawberry stand filled with those big red berries.

I loved working with the youngsters who were between the ages of 12 and 16. Maybe our area has been specially blessed, but most of the young people I've worked with year after year came from a mold of the highest caliber.

During September, we plowed and disced the 100 acres of harvested oat ground along with some additional fallow ground, and planted 170 acres to winter wheat, completely unaware of how far that wheat crop would eventually take us.

In October, Dr. John Nesbitt carefully examined this diabetic woman of 26 years, giving me an excellent report at the end of the examination. I must say, I liked the young doctor immediately.

Without our cows to care for, the cabbage and corn harvest progressed rapidly. My husband taught me how to operate our newly purchased grain dryer. When the corn was dried and cooled, it flowed from the dryer into an elevator which deposited the corn into a grain bin.

After the harvest was completed, my husband concentrated his efforts on getting our farm machinery ready for the next planting season, along with the constant process of marketing our grains. I again invested my extra energies into that never ending job of record keeping.

It was a great feeling, however, to pull the covers back over my head on those cold, snowy mornings and no longer worry about trudging to the barn.

At the December meeting of the Conneaut School Board, my husband was elected president, a position he would hold for the next four years.

That winter Willy and I spent some time leafing through travel brochures. We both wanted to visit Western Europe. In March we decided on a 16-day vacation the following August with Successful Farming's tour department. Successful Farming publishes a farm magazine. Their travel itinerary highlighted exactly what we wanted to see.

It was lovely planning that vacation so far ahead. It allowed me plenty of time to dream while accomplishing jobs to help with the spring planting.

In July, Willy joyfully harvested a bumper crop of wheat from the 170 acres planted the preceeding year.

On August 2, after leaving John in the care of my mother, Willy and I drove to Cleveland, Ohio, to begin the first leg of our European vacation. At the airport we were introduced to two young couples from Ohio, and a single young man from Michigan who would also be taking the same trip. After only a few minutes of conversation together, we felt like we had known each other all our lives.

Everyone is a bit apprehensive when traveling abroad for the first time, and although we had been to Hawaii, you could hardly call us seasoned travelers. However, this was the first trip any of our new friends had taken, so we bonded together like peas in a pod.

Our flight to New York was delayed because of severe thunderstorms over that city, but we were in such good company we paid little attention to the time.

We were scheduled to board a British Airways flight at nine o'clock that evening in New York. But it's only a hop, skip, and a jump from Cleveland to New York or so we thought.

Finally, at five thirty that evening, we boarded the airplane headed for New York. We still had plenty of time to catch our flight, but after reaching New York, our airplane was put in the all too familiar holding pattern over the John F. Kennedy airport. After 45 minutes in this pattern the pilot announced that we were going to land at the Bethlehem-Easton airport in Allentown, Pennsylvania, to take on fuel. It was then we heard a woman's pitiful moan behind us saying, "Oh no, we're out of fuel!"

It was almost too funny for words. Each person that overheard the remark tried to console her. But her husband said it best, while patting her shaking hand, "Honey, you just have to trust the pilot."

"Oh, how true," I thought, "Not only when flying, but trusting our Pilot through life as well."

We did land safely, and after taking on fuel, resumed our place in the holding pattern while still on the ground until given clearance for a straight-in approach landing.

However, our plenty of time to catch the next flight had run out. After landing at J.F.K. Airport, everyone was late. You should have seen the people dashing out of that 737. The stewardess could have been crushed.

This was our first time at Kennedy Airport. We could easily see the British Airways terminal, but it was too far for us to walk. We tried to hail a taxi, but when we told them where we wanted to go, they refused to take us. We later realized that the British Airways terminal was only a $3.00 run for them. Had we been smart, and held up a $20.00 bill, we could have made it by taxi.

Being unseasoned travelers, we did the next best thing and hopped the shuttle bus which only runs one way, requiring us to make a complete loop around the terminal.

While riding the shuttle, we chatted with a British couple who were headed for the same flight we were. What luck! They were seasoned travelers. When we climbed off the shuttle they knew exactly where to go. We followed them up a staircase where a woman walked out of an office, and hollered, "They're here!"

She was the guide our group was supposed to meet at Kennedy Airport. Then, we heard a woman inside the office talking to our pilot, who had started out, but was not yet on the runway.

"He'll bring the plane back!" Our guide announced happily. Minutes later, we entered a 747 where people were already sprawled out half asleep. We missed the safety instructions, but were grateful we didn't miss our plane.

It took a while to wind down after all that excitement. I'm quite sure no one slept much that night. We were all too busy chatting. Just a few short hours together, and we had, indeed, formed lifelong friendships.

A travel agent met us at Heathrow Airport in London, England, and escorted us to our hotel. It was a beautiful, sunny morning and the balance of our day was free to rest or explore London on our own.

I'd tested my urine, and taken my insulin injection in the tiny Ladies' room aboard the airplane (not an easy feat) shortly before they served breakfast. So, after a short rest, Willy and I met with our new friends, and together took a double-decker bus ride combined with shopping. When we exited the final store, everyone except my husband had lost their sense of direction. However, he's been especially blessed with a keen one, and he guided us to the correct bus for our ride back to the hotel.

Baggage transfer was provided on our tour, but due to our late arrival at the New York airport, our luggage did not get off the airplane when we did. I'm sure I don't have to remind you never to pack your insulin and syringes in your suitcase when traveling!

Incidentally, I was a little hesitant of traveling abroad with insulin syringes in my purse, so I carried a note from my doctor stating that I was an insulin-dependent diabetic. I never needed to show that note to anyone, but if there had been any question while going through the boarding gates, I was prepared.

We spent three days in London, visiting

the Parliament Building, Westminister Abby, St. Paul's Cathedral, and Trafalgar Square. We saw many landmarks, including Big Ben and the changing of the guards at Buckingham Palace.

Ours, being a farm tour allowed us the opportunity to visit a farm involved in hybrid hog production. We took a scenic drive close to Wales. I fell in love with Anne Hathaway's cottage and marveled at the peaceful gravesite of Sr. Winston Churchill near the village church of Bladon in Oxfordshire.

Eventually, we boarded a Comet jet for our flight to Holland. My husband is six feet tall. We were packed into that airplane so tight he could not move his feet. The Comet jet was not near as spacious as the newer jets.

Everyone was glad to get off that airplane and into the air-conditioned motor coach our tour guide, Nels Neilson, had waiting for us.

We toured Amsterdam, taking a launch trip along some of the quaint canals. We stopped at a Fishing village and were fascinated by the Zuider Zee, which was once the largest bay in the Netherlands, but is being continually drained to add acres of farm land to that country. I was surprised to learn that the rest of the Zuider Zee has been changed from salt water to fresh water and is known as Lake Eisel.

Driving past Dutch farms into Germany, we visited Cologne where we toured a magnificent cathedral. The Deutz tractor people also treated us to a delicious lunch at their International Headquarters.

It's difficult to remember all the places we saw; however, one thing we will never forget is the wonderful people we met on that trip.

Everyone fell in love with our tour guide.

If I could only remember half the information he gave us, I would be a walking encyclopedia.

From Germany we traveled through the corner of Austria and into the tiny country of Lichtenstein on our way to the lovely lakeside resort of Lucerne, Switzerland.

The following day I declined a trip up Mt. Platus, where my husband and Louie (the single young man from Michigan) rode a ski lift and cable car to the top of the mountain, and a cog railroad train back down.

When they described the view, along with the faint tinkle of cow bells ascending up that mountain, I realized I'd missed a great adventure. But I wanted more shopping time and found a store named Bucherer, which is the largest watch and jewelry retailer in Switzerland. How could anyone travel to Switzerland without purchasing a Swiss watch or two?

Well, the truth is, I bought more than two and purchased several cuckoo clocks to be shipped to some of our friends and relatives back in the states.

From Lucerne we traveled to Zurich, where we toured a newspaper publisher's farm, which was a combination dairy and hog farm. Most naturally the cattle were Brown Swiss.

I'm glad I did not have to choose a favorite country from those we visited because it would have been quite impossible for me to do so. As we motored towards Vichy, France, I sadly realized our vacation would soon be ending.

We spent only twenty-four hours in Vichy and from there we headed for our final destination, Paris.

Our guide, Nels Neilson, was a Norwegian. He was a bit more than bilingual, having the ability to speak five languages quite fluently. He could also imitate anyone's voice near perfectly. Our young son loved to watch Hogan's Heroes on television back then. When we called home from Paris, Nels imitated Colonel Klink's voice so perfectly, that for a quick moment I almost forgot who he was. To our disappointment John wasn't fooled . . . or so he says.

That evening we dined in the Eiffel Tower, surveying the lights of Paris. The following day we visited the Arc de Triumphe, Notre Dame, and the Louvre, to name just a few. And, of course, I visited some lovely Paris dress shops.

It was midnight when our airplane finally touched down in Cleveland, Ohio, and after one o'clock the following morning before we checked into the Holiday Inn in that city. It had been twenty-six hours since we got up in Paris, France, that morning. You can believe we were two tired people, but filled with the pleasant memories of a splendid vacation.

Mother listened with fascination as I described our trip.

"Now that you've done that you must take a cruise, it's such a wonderful way to travel," She exclaimed.

Each winter she and her friends would "get together" for a Caribbean Cruise. She really loved sailing and her description of life on board a cruise ship made me tingle with excitement!

In late August mother went to spend some time with Ida, but before leaving, she urged me to bring my family to Florida that winter for a Caribbean Cruise.

During the next several weeks our family

discussed different vacation options we might want to consider in the future. One evening I suggested a Caribbean Cruise.

"Well," my husband replied, "I'd like to see a little more than the Caribbean."

Now, I really wasn't for or against the Caribbean, I just wanted to take a cruise.

Later that fall Willy started keeping a close eye on the grain futures, hoping to move some of our bountiful wheat crop to market. He checked the Wall Street Journal faithfully, as he did everyday, but with a special eye trained on the market. As the cash price moved up, he shipped several trailer loads of the nutritious grain.

Our corn and cabbage harvest was now in full swing. David Naas, a young man who had worked several summers for us, graduated from high school and was now employed full time completely handling the grain drying operation, while I worked in the cabbage field.

Willy was again harvesting corn day and night. And it was up to me to keep an eye on the wheat market.

One evening while thumbing through the Wall Street Journal, I ran across a half-page advertisement from the Cunard Steamship Company, announcing their maiden round-the-world voyage of the Queen Elizabeth 2. It listed the ports of call along with prices, and this invitation:

> January 4th 1975 will be a proud day for Cunard. On that day, the greatest ship in the world is due to set sail on her first round the world voyage, at the same time making history.

Queen Elizabeth 2 will visit five continents, and cross three oceans. It will be the first time since the War that Cunard have undertaken a world cruise from Southhampton. So I am excited to offer you this opportunity to sail with us.

Because she's much faster than the average cruise ship, the QE2 will be calling at many more ports; 23 in all. From Bombay in India to Balboa in Panama, Cape Town in South Africa to Colombo in Ceylon.

Truly the voyage of a lifetime.

In between ports you'll cruise in the absolute luxury you would expect from us. The QE2 is a magnificent ship. Her accommodation rivals the best hotels and in service we aim for perfection. Our cuisine, we believe, can create the finest food at sea.

In port we'll look after you with as much care as when on the QE2. For the last two decades American Express have set high standards in arranging shore excursions for Cunard. We have asked them to do so again for this occasion. So you'll have the opportunity to tour every country that we visit.

I invite you to join us on this historic occasion. This, above all, will be the voyage to remember.

When I finished reading the advertisement, I clipped it from the newspaper, and placed it on our kitchen table where my husband would be sure to see it when he walked in the door.

Now I really did it for a joke! However, he still refuses to believe it. Later that evening while I refilled his thermos, he picked up the advertisement studying it carefully.

"How's that for a cruise?" I asked with a chuckle.

He responded with his famous grin, saying, "why don't you send for the brochure?"

You probably won't be surprised to learn that the letter I typed to Cunard requesting their brochure could have been entered in the Guinness Book of Records as the fastest letter ever typed.

After receiving the brochure, my husband and I were very interested. He contacted the New York office of Cunard Lines, where, after a number of telephone calls over a period of several weeks, Cunard reserved a room for us on their maiden round-the-world voyage.

Our next step was to talk to John's fifth grade school teacher about this trip. His response was overwhelming.

"He'll learn more on that trip than he will in my classroom," He remarked. He also would provide a study outline for John to follow as we promised to teach him the required subjects.

As we walked towards the classroom door he commented, "Could you find room in your suitcase for me?"

How well I understood his request for it still seemed unbelievable that we were really going on this trip.

When things settled down, I realized I'd truly have to hustle to ever be ready in time. It seemed like such a huge undertaking. We were scheduled to board the ship in New York City on Friday, January 10, and would be returning home on Monday, March 31.

The first item on our agenda was securing

the proper vaccinations. On the morning of November 5, we went to the State Health Department in Erie for our yellow fever vaccination, and in the afternoon to Dr. Kirkpatrick's office in Meadville for a smallpox and cholera vaccination.

We returned home to load a final truck with cabbage. When my husband looked up he had a hard time seeing the road. Also, at a school board meeting later that evening, he had a difficult time seeing the people in the back of the room.

Willy was experiencing a reaction to one of the vaccinations. But I want you to know they never phased me at all.

At times I've heard the remark: "Oh, I couldn't possibly do that," made by insulin-dependent diabetics regarding different opportunities in life. It is a remark I hate to hear because you and I are capable of doing anything we want to do . . . it's all up to us.

In December, my husband cash contracted the balance of our wheat crop at an excellent price, with delivery scheduled within 30 days. This is precisely what every farmer dreams about. A good price for an abundant crop.

> Oh that men would praise the Lord for his goodness, and for his wonderful works to the children of men.
>
> For he satisfieth the longing soul and filleth the hungry soul with goodness.
>
> Psalm 107:8,9.

CHAPTER 12

The Dream of a Lifetime

At 12:15 on the morning of January 10, 1975, Willy, John, and myself, boarded a Greyhound Bus in Pittsburgh, Pennsylvania, with nine suitcases and three carryon cases. I'd been packing for several weeks and now that the strain of preparing for this vacation was behind me, I relaxed in my seat. However, I was much too excited to sleep. While my eyes viewed the night scenery, my mind tried to fathom just what was in store for us.

We arrived in New York City shortly after 7:00 that morning, and while Willy and John gathered our luggage, I hurried to the Ladies' room of the bus station, where I tested my urine and took my insulin injection. During our taxi ride to the dock, I ate a small snack knowing breakfast would be delayed.

How exciting New York City is! Soon, our taxi pulled up to the dock where a porter took our luggage while we stared in amazement at the monstrous vessel which was going to be our home for the next 80 days. It's hard to describe a ship, but she looked absolutely beautiful to us.

Actually, we were not permitted to board the ship until five o'clock that evening. Knowing this, we planned to show John as much of New York City as we possibly could before boarding. Our muscles were still stiff from riding, so after breakfast on the wharf, we walked the ten blocks uptown, stopping at Rockefeller Center.

We'd given the porter our luggage, but never surrendered our carry on cases. My husband shouldered the heavy ones filled with cameras and film, while I tucked the case with my diabetic supplies carefully under my arm.

Willy sunburns easily, so he purchased a Stetson hat, with the broad brim, and high soft crown to protect him on this trip. Rather than pack it he wore it. When we stepped inside Sac's 5th Avenue, a saleslady definitely thought he was from Australia. How disappointed she was when we assured her he was "only" from Pennsylvania.

After touring and lunch at the United Nations Building, we boarded the subway for a trip to the Statue of Liberty. After visiting the statue our afternoon slipped away. Returning uptown by subway, we again hailed a taxi which took us to Pier 48 where we boarded the magnificent ship.

Our luggage was in our stateroom when we arrived and my several weeks of packing was unpacked in thirty minutes.

The Queen Elizabeth 2 had 29 grades of air-conditioned staterooms to choose from, each with ample wardrobe space, as well as private bathrooms with all facilities. All staterooms had regular beds, no upper berths, complete with radio and telephone, and ours, room number 4148, was very comfortable.

There were three restaurants on board: The Britannia, the Columbia, and the Queen's Grill. Each days three main meals were served at leisurely single sittings. Also available each day was mid-morning bouillon, afternoon tea and pastries, and a sumptuous midnight buffet. That first evening we were cordially escorted to our table in the warmly decorated Britannia Restaurant.

Each table was served by at least three waiters. A smiling, happy young man named Arnie, informed us that he would be our chief waiter throughout the cruise.

The menu was elegant, filled with excellent choices including plenty of salads, fresh vegetables, and a fine selection of fresh fruit, truly an exceptional menu for any diabetic to choose from. After an excellent dinner we waited excitedly for the ship's departure.

At last the majestic horn sounded and the ship set sail. How impressive the Statue of Liberty looked. The Verrazano-Narrows bridge was quite a sight as we crossed under it. The New York skyline was also fantastic. It was midnight when we finally climbed into bed after a long, exciting day.

It was a bit rocky when we awoke the following morning. But after a delightful breakfast, we dallied at our table watching the waves tumble.

Then we decided to explore our new home. Since virtually all of this cruise would be through Equatorial or near Equatorial climates, we could look forward to substantial open-deck activity. Six of the ship's decks had open areas. Two decks each had outdoor swimming pools with every deck sport you could imagine available.

For those to whom the sun was less friendly, the ship also provided two indoor pools, a complete gymnasium, sauna, turkish bath, and massage room along with a cinema and game room.

The personal services included complete laundry and dry cleaning services, two laundrettes, barbering and hairstyling salons, facilities for church services, along with a bank, post office, a complete shopping center, and a fully equipped hospital as well as dental services. She was truly a city at sea.

Mortimer Hehir, was then captain of the QE2. He had a distinguished record since first joining Cunard Line in 1937 as third officer on the cargo ship Bantria. In 1942 he obtained his Master's Ticket in Liverpool and was sent to join the Queen Elizabeth, which was operating a regular troup-carrying run from New York to Greenock, Scotland. In 1970 he joined the QE2 as staff captain, and in 1973, following the retirement of its present captain, Mortimer Hehir succeeded as master of the QE2.

The deck space of the spacious ship was 4500 square yards, one of the largest of any passenger ship in the world. Ten of her thirteen decks were devoted to passengers.

She was also the first passenger vessel equipped to navigate by space satellite. Her receiving equipment enabled her to pick up signals transmitted by satellites, orbiting the earth 600 miles up.

Her computer system was the first of its kind in a Merchant Ship. It combined technical, operational, and commercial functions while at sea. These included data logging, alarm scanning, machinery control, weather routing, the prediction of fresh water requirements, and the control of food stocks on board.

Incidentally, she could also carry 6413 tons of fuel oil. Her rudder weighed 80 tons, and her four anchors weighed 12-1/2 tons each with cables up to 2200 feet long. Her gross tonnage was 66,000 tons.

If you ever referred to her as a boat, you risked being thrown overboard. She was a ship, of course, in the very finest sense of the word.

After learning all this, we spent our first day aboard ship quite in awe of our new home away from home.

On our second morning out of New York, we could see the Florida coastline while eating breakfast. Later, we watched in fascination as our ship picked up a pilot from a pilot boat and two accompanying tug boats guided us safely into the harbor at Port Everglades, Florida. Likewise, we would watch this event time after time with great fascination as pilots and tugs the world around guided the massive ship into their harbor.

We spent only five hours in Port Everglades, just long enough to take on passengers. We spent our time visiting with mother and her friends who had come to see the massive ship.

How disappointed we were when she could

not tour the ship. But security on board was especially tight for this maiden voyage and passenger's guests were not permitted on board.

After bidding farewell to Florida, our ship skirted the Carribbean, docking at Curacao in the Netherlands, Antilles, a group of islands not far off the coast of South America.

Oil refining is the major industry of the islands, and as the ship approached, we could see refinery fires in the distance. We had seven hours to see the sights. I'm quite sure our ship took on fuel the entire seven hours.

Willemstad, the capital, was a charming town, full of quaint gabled houses, unmistakably Dutch. Our tour guide was excellent, and after touring, Willy and I shopped for bargains in this fabulous freeport while John went back to the ship to swim.

We always booked tours in advance with American Express whose office was in easy reach aboard ship. However, our greatest help with touring came from Mr. William Harris, a world traveler many times over who provided informative lectures before each port-of-call, allowing us to choose the more significant sights from his recommendations. He also advised us on the more favorable purchases available in each country.

Before leaving Pennsylvania, I specifically stocked up on insulin, syringes and clinitest tablets. I also had a good supply of vitamin B12 along. Remember, when traveling extensively it is extremely important for us to do this. Extra . . . is always the rule of thumb.

En route from Curacao, the Queen made her first of five Equatorial crossings, which were celebrated with traditional ceremony. Everyone within reach of the swimming pool got dumped in including our John. Some got slathered with ketchup before landing there. When the fun was over, the swimming pool was a gory mess.

Salvador was our first port-of-call in South America, the capital of Bahia, one of the nine states of Brazil. It looked beautiful from the ship. After anchoring in the bay we traveled to shore by launch, which in itself was a great experience.

Our tour took us to magnificent baroque churches, along with old forts, and picturesque markets. This area is the part of South America which is nearest to Africa. African influences were evident throughout the city.

On January 22, we viewed the enchanting Rio de Janeiro Harbor entrance. It was cloudy, but fantastic. That morning we rode a cable car up Sugar Loaf Mountain.

We also visited Corcovados Pinnacle, 2300 feet above sea level, which brought us to the giant statue of Christ. And in the afternoon, journeyed to Sterns, where we watched beautiful stones being made into jewelry.

That evening, we talked to David Naas from the ship's telephone. David was busy keeping a close watch on the farm while we were gone.

The following day we started across the Southern Atlantic Ocean headed for Cape Town, South Africa. About a day before arriving in Cape Town, our captain announced that the ocean depth where we were sailing was three miles deep. Almost unbelievable!

But by this time Willy was having a tough

time keeping his sea legs under him. When we got to Cape Town, I'm sure he would have walked, if there had been a 4-lane highway, home.

The real truth is the harbor entrance into Cape Town is so narrow that the ship was held out a day due to 40 MPH winds. After docking, we ambled along oak-shaded lanes and cobbled streets, touring the Botanical Gardens where wild flowers cover the slopes of Table Mountain.

After enjoying Cape Town's hospitality, we sailed 800 miles around the Cape of Good Hope to Durban. Here our tour took us into the Valley of 1,000 Hills, which is a vast Zulu reserve, to Natal Lion Park. We then passed through beautiful rugged mountain scenery, where wild game is preserved in the park in a natural setting. While in the reserve, we glimpsed the Zulu's way of life and watched as they performed native dances.

While sailing from Durban to Mombasa, representatives of the Cunard Steamship Company gave each round-the-world passenger a lovely silver medallion. Engraved on one side was each port-of-call, and on the other, a picture of the beautiful ship. A truly memorable gift from a never to be forgotten vacation.

What was life really like on board this vessel? Words like wonderful, incredible, and fantastic, come close to describing this worry free vacation. But aside from the impeccable quality of life on board ship, the wonderful people we met were indeed its crowning glory.

John discovered a complete family of aunts, uncles, grandmothers, and grandfathers on board. After the lovely Lillian Gish signed his autograph book, she invited him to have lunch with her. He accepted, of course. I only hope he remembered his manners.

When we reached Mombasa, John and his dad took a 2-day safari into Tsavo Park West staying overnight at Ngulia Safari Lodge. They saw every wild animal imaginable. John talked about it for days.

I chose to stay on board ship. When my family left, I immediately put on my "I am a diabetic" necklace. Then, I spent a day in Tsavo Park East, enjoying a luncheon at Voi Safari Lodge with friends, whom I had previously informed about my diabetes.

From Mombasa we sailed to the Seychelles, an island infrequently visited by outsiders. They are sometimes called the Forgotten Islands. Yet this drowsy, dream-like island group in the Indian Ocean has been called the most beautiful on earth.

The principal island is Mahe, where we rode a glass bottomed boat to see the coral gardens. The heat and humidity were high, but the flowers and coconut palms were especially beautiful.

As we docked in Bombay, India, the tugboat pilot used a megaphone, rather than a 2-way radio to communicate with our captain on the bridge.

We spent four days in that country. John and his dad flew to Delhi, where sightseeing included the Parliament and Government Buildings. Tours in Old Delhi also included the Red Fort and the Birla Temple.

The following morning they flew to the "Pink City" of Jaipur, and drove to the ancient capital of Amber for an exciting elephant ride to its Hillside

Palace. In the afternoon they saw the Palace of the Winds, along with Maharajah's Cenotaphs. That evening they flew to Agra.

Before daylight the next morning they stood at the Taj Mahal, watching the sun as it poured every color imaginable over the marble dome minarets, truly a breathtaking sight. Later, they drove to the deserted city of Fatehpur Sikri, the ancient capital city of palaces, which was abandoned by the moghuls at the end of the 16th century.

Their flight back to Bombay was delayed, however, and it was the middle of the night before the group returned to the ship. Everyone, including me, of course, was worried sick. And the stress involved warranted a close watch of my blood sugar. Nevertheless, when they finally returned, telling of their wonderful adventure, all worry was forgotten.

Once again I chose to stay on board ship, taking advantage of several day long tours in Bombay, desperately seeking to broaden my knowledge of that impoverished country.

Leaving India, we sailed to Sr. Lanka, the new name for Ceylon, and found the capital, Colombo, one of the busiest centers in the East. If you ever visit that country, don't miss the elephant performance at the Colombo Zoo. It is known the world over and it is delightful.

From Ceylon we continued across the Indian Ocean, through the Straits of Malacca into Singapore, where among other attractions we toured the "Tiger Balm" gardens, a sort of Eastern Disneyland, with caves, grottos, and painted mythological statues.

After sailing on the Queen, I realized sailors aren't "made," they are "born." It takes a special love of the sea to enlist a man in that profession.

We often sailed for days at a time without ever sighting land only occasionally passing a freighter at sea. However, I must admit, I especially loved those days when there was only the sea and sky with which to contend. It was during that time my thoughts sometimes drifted back to my youth and Dr. Stoney. Oh, how I wished he were still alive, so that I could thank him for giving me the formula to live successfully with my diabetes.

Likewise, in the evening, the galaxy of stars were beautiful! Almost within reach, and many times I focused my thoughts on the following Psalm:

> When I consider thy heavens,
> the work of thy fingers, the moon
> and stars which thou hast
> ordained.
> What is man, that thou dost
> take thought of him? And the
> Son of man, that thou dost care
> for him?
> Yet Thou hast made him a little
> lower than God, and dost crown
> him with glory and majesty!
> Thou dost make him to rule over
> the works of thy hands. Thou
> hast put all things under his
> feet.
> All sheep and oxen and also the
> beasts of the field.
> The birds of the heavens, and
> the fish of the sea, whatever
> passes through the paths of the
> sea.

> Oh Lord our Lord. How majestic
> is thy name in all the earth!
>
> Psalm 8.

Consequently, on that vacation I experienced a new appreciation of God's infinite provision for man.

On February 22, our view from the ship was magnificent as we sailed towards the lovely island of Bali. Bali was indeed a magical island of deserted beaches, tropical forests, and lush paddy fields. The people were strikingly attractive, and they, as well as the island, were as yet unspoiled by commercialization or mass tourism. Bali was definitely my favorite spot.

Threading her way north through the islands of the East Indies, our ship sailed towards Hong Kong for a 4-day visit. We were up early to watch the approach into Victoria Harbor. Here, aged junks with patched sails, were dwarfed by giant freighters, along with tiny water taxis and fishing boats. There was feverish activity everywhere!

Our very first evening in Hong Kong was spent with Doris Chan, a remarkable woman we met on board ship. She took twenty-two of us to the Very Good Restaurant for a "real" Chinese dinner.

The following morning we toured the New Territories, looking across into Red China, experiencing a new appreciation for our beloved freedom. And of course, we shopped in a glittering array of tiny stores, packed together with brightly painted signs.

On March 5, we docked in the busy harbor at Kobe, Japan, and while walking, spotted a familiar sight: a McDonald's Restaurant.

While in Kobe we toured Kyoto, visiting the Heian Shrine, the Gold Pavilion, and Nijo Castle, with its famous "nightingale" floors, which sing to you as you step on them.

The following day was bright and sunny as we docked at Yokohama. Mount Fugi, so often covered with clouds, was a beautiful sight.

Did you know that diabetes is also prevalent in Japan? In addition, there is increased speculation that if a break-through ever occurs, it will probably originate in this country.

Surprisingly though, this was one of the two countries in which we experienced language difficulties. Some of the young Japanese speak English, but we were very much "on our own" when not on tour.

Our experience purchasing tickets for an Express Train ride was a bit confusing, but we did manage to get to Tokyo, where we visited the Imperial Palace and the Diet Building, to name a few. However, while we admired the sights of Japan, the Japanese people marveled at the sight of the QE2. They flocked day and night to see this magnificent ship docked in their harbor.

We were now headed across the Pacific towards Honolulu, Hawaii, and on that segment, we crossed the International Date Line.

Passing over the date line is a timeless moment. For it is where our days begin and end, simultaneously. The date line is imaginary, drawn north and south largely along the 180th meridian, passing between Siberia and Alaska in the north, and between Ellice Island and Somoa further south.

It is along this line that all the nations of the world have agreed that each calendar day will begin at midnight. So that when it is Sunday just west of the line, it is still Saturday east of it. And as we crossed from west to east, we bid goodbye to today, and hello to yesterday.

When we docked in Honolulu it was cloudy, but beautiful, as the Hawaiian Band played the National Anthem. We were only in port a few hours. For a change of pace we enjoyed lunch at the Sheraton Waikiki.

On Wednesday, March 19, after five days at sea, we docked at Los Angeles where we spent the day at Disneyland. This was my first visit to California and I loved it.

From Los Angeles we sailed to Acapulco, where after dropping anchor we again took a launch to shore. We spent the day on the beach watching people ski, kite fly, and sky dive. A remarkable sight. And of course, we shopped.

This was truly a wonderful way to travel. In each and every country, we could always count on the same comfortable bed to sleep in at night.

Likewise, it was perfect for me knowing my insulin was safe in the hospital refrigerator. But while this was the ultimate in vacations as far as I was concerned, I was very careful not to vacation from my diabetic control plan which would have been foolish. Although sometimes it was a bit difficult. Nevertheless, I carefully managed my insulin, exercise, and eating so I could truly enjoy this trip.

On March 25, we entered the port of Balboa at the entrance to the Panama Canal. We were up at dawn so we could get a good spot to watch from on the front deck and in fascination, watched our ship navigate the Rio Grande, and enter the Miraflores Locks, to rise 54 feet above sea level into Miraflores Lake. Electrically-driven mules hauled the giant ship through the locks to avoid unnecessary pressure.

Further down, locks lifted the ship into Gillard Cut, a narrow eight mile stretch, which is constantly dredged to keep the channel clear. Then into Gatun Lake, One Hundred-Sixty miles of inland water, held in check by a huge dam 85 feet above sea level. From there our descent began, through a series of three locks, each with two compartments that allows two ships to pass through simultaneously in opposite directions. It took the ship eight hours to transit the canal; but what a sight!

When we looked at each other, we were also a sight. We had watched our ship transit the canal in total fascination not realizing how hot the sun was. And Willy and I got a dilly of a sunburn. (What a dumb thing for a diabetic to do)!

The following morning we anchored at Cartagena, Colombia. This turned out to be the hottest day of our entire trip. Willy and I walked into town, this time slathered in suntan lotion (better late than never) and visited several landmarks. In addition, Cartagena was also the second country in which we experienced some problems communicating.

Soon, our ship glided into Kingston, Jamaica, an island south of Cuba in the West Indies. Whenever I think of Kingston, I'll always remember the Straw Market which featured innumerable items made from straw.

Two days later, we again docked in Port Everglades, Florida, to unload passengers. Yes, our wonderful vacation was finally winding down. After church services that Easter Sunday in March, we spent our final day as we had so many days with the wonderful people that made this vacation so special.

Finally, on March 31, the huge ship pulled into New York harbor where we disembarked. Getting through customs with all our purchases was a real experience! Then, we packed the three of us and our now eighteen pieces of luggage into a rented car for our trip back to Pennsylvania.

In spite of the fact that my husband experienced a rough beginning, he will invariably tell you he would never have missed that superb vacation.

After a trip like that, even the most tedious jobs seemed easy, and the rest of that year just glided by. The strong grain prices we were then enjoying allowed us to purchase a new Gleaner combine for harvesting our grains.

Recently, the Albro Packing Company in Springboro had been sold to another company. That company in turn sold the kraut and pickle works to an individual. Rumors were now flying about the financial stability of this new owner.

In April of 1976, Willy and I flew to San Francisco for a National School Board Convention. Willy was busy attending a variety of seminars. I spent my time with Mrs. Paavola, another school board member's wife from Erie.

Mrs. Paavola knew San Francisco well, and she showed me most of the sights including the exquisite shops on Fisherman's Wharf.

During the last leg of that journey, our return flight from Pittsburgh to Erie, the plane was crowded. After landing, we hurried to exit, when two men from the back of the airplane began hollering John's name.

He greeted them, and when we reached the airport, they hustled him into a corner jabbering non-stop.

I stood in amazement watching these men, who had cornered my husband, and now had him engaged in a captive conversation. In a few minutes, the men started smiling and shook hands with Willy. After bidding them goodbye, he stepped over to where I was standing, exclaiming:

"Those men are the new owners of the Albro. They want us to sign a contract for 1500 tons of cabbage this year!"

Wow! I could hardly believe my ears. From the rumors circulating we thought cabbage was a thing of the past. But this sounded wonderful and the price they offered was excellent.

The following day one of the men appeared at our door with a contract for my husband to sign.

During that planting season we worked feverishly, trying to get forty acres of kraut cabbage set along with all our other farm work. When we finally succeeded we took a complete rest.

Willy, John, and I boarded a 747 in New York City, for a sixteen day vacation into some of the Scandinavian countries.

Reaching Denmark, we spent two days in Copenhagen, and from there, took a ferry trip to Jonkoping, Sweden, where we rode a most scenic highway into Stockholm and Karlstad, marveling at the beauty of each country.

After touring Karlstad we entered Lille-hammer, Norway, and visited Elvester, passing through Fjord country into Tyin. We continued through the lovely Norwegian lake country to Fager-ness, then onto Oslo.

From Oslo we boarded an overnight steamer, returning us to Denmark for our flight back to London where we showed John as many sights as we could before flying home.

In September, our strawberries began sprouting a few too many weeds. I decided to remove them before they went to seed for the winter. One warm day while I was busily engaged in that task, my husband drove in, walked up the row to where I was working. When I looked up at him, I knew something was terribly wrong!

"I've got some bad news," he said grimly. He then informed me that the man who held our 1500-ton cabbage contract had just filed for bankruptcy, and we were stuck with 40 acres of kraut cabbage with no market.

What a blow!

Fortunately, however, the cash market was strong that year, and cabbage in New York was scarce because of an extremely wet planting season. Several days later a man from New York stopped at our farm, looking for enough cabbage to fill his companies' requirement. As a result, what could have been a sub-stantial loss for us turned out to be a much needed crop indeed. That experience taught us never to under-estimate the power of supply and demand.

That fall we worked steadily, cutting and loading cabbage into semi-trailers for the trip to New York.

As the cabbage harvest was winding down, I took a day off to clean the house and do some much needed baking. Early that morning I kneaded a huge glob of bread dough. While it was raising, I polished the house until it glowed.

When I popped the bread in the oven early that afternoon, I was exhausted. After the 10-minute timer rang, I transferred the top and bottom loaves around so they would brown evenly, turned the oven temperature down, set the timer for an additional 30 minutes, and collapsed into a living room chair.

No problem, I thought, I'll just rest a few minutes while that bread is baking, and then I'll be good as new. However, when I finally awoke, I was trying to converse with my husband, who was offering me orange juice with sugar.

John had come home from school that afternoon and found me unconscious, still in the chair soaked through with sweat. He quickly ran to fetch his dad.

When Willy reached me, he immediately recognized a severe insulin reaction. He placed me carefully on the carpeted floor, covered me, then, mixed an injection of Glucagon, and administered it.

In a short time I regained consciousness.

"Oh no," I moaned, "I've got bread in the oven!"

Willy helped me unload the bread, which did not burn, but instead, turned hard as a rock. After the bread cooled, my husband sawed through a loaf and took half of it out for our dog, Lady, to gnaw on. But much to our dismay she wouldn't touch it.

Smart dog!

Consequently, my ten loaves of homemade

bread went into the garbage.

What a hard lesson to learn. You would think that now, after 30 years as an insulin-dependent diabetic, I would never get caught in a mess like that. But somehow, I've never reached a plateau in my diabetic management plan, where I can safely relax my control like I did that day. And I am quite certain I never will.

CHAPTER 13

The Eyes Have It

In mid-January of 1977, my husband and I attended a 2-day seminar on strawberry production at the Hershey Motor Lodge in Hershey, Pennsylvania. This again, was sponsored by the Pennsylvania State University. We usually try to attend these meetings together, because our farming operation is a combined effort.

The first day of meetings was very informative and we met strawberry growers from all over the state. We now had 10 acres of the delightful fruit under cultivation. Besides excellent speakers, growers could also gain helpful information from each other through explicit grower inter-action. At this particular meeting, we were introduced to a man, probably in his early sixties, who was raising some 20 acres of strawberries in Eastern Pennsylvania.

He sat with Willy and me at the session following lunch that first day, and the next morning he again slipped in beside us. He seemed like such a nice man. I wondered if he might be a widower, but following the afternoon session, he asked us to save a seat for him and his wife at the banquet that evening which would conclude the seminar.

Our friend looked quite solemn when talking about his wife, saying she was ill, and had not been feeling good enough to attend the sessions. While dressing for dinner that evening, I couldn't help but feel a stab of pity for the nice man and his sickly wife.

The dining room filled rapidly, and we had a difficult time trying to save two seats for our friend. Finally, he and his wife appeared and she sat down beside me.

Soon, the preliminary greeting started, and while our host was speaking, I wondered what could possibly be wrong with the woman sitting beside me.

However, I didn't have to wait long to find out, because she leaned towards me while our dinner was being served, and began telling me all her troubles.

During the past year she had really been sick, and when she described her illness, it sounded dreadful! She even had to take some kind of terrible injection each day.

Finally, because I could hardly stand the suspense, I turned towards her waiting to hear the name of this illness.

She again leaned towards me, and with her eyes rolled slightly upwards, announced: "I'm a diabetic!"

For a moment I sat stunned, not wanting to believe what I was hearing. However, as she continued talking about her terrible illness, I suddenly wanted to laugh. Then, after listening to her, I decided I wanted to cry, not so much for her, but for the dear man sitting beside her. This couple was nearing their retirement years, which should have been a satisfying time. But she was now criticizing her husband for continuing his healthy farming operation while she was ailing.

Finally, I'd heard enough, and I turned towards the woman saying, "I've been an insulin-dependent diabetic for 30 years."

"You!" She exclaimed and this time her eyes rolled all the way up in her head. "But you look so healthy."

"I am healthy," I replied, "and you can be too." However, by this time the speaker had been introduced. And she hurriedly excused herself without listening to what I was saying.

As she made her exit, she muttered, "I must go back to the room, I really feel better when I'm laying down."

That evening, I didn't hear much of what the speaker was saying, because my eyes kept glancing at the dear man one seat away. He looked weary and my heart went out to him.

Its been 10 years since that happened, but the memory is still clearly etched in my mind. Every time I think of that woman, I'm reminded of the story of Nicolo Paganini, the gifted violinist.

Paganini was standing before a packed house, playing a magnificent piece of music while the orchestra offered a majestic accompaniment, when suddenly, one string on Paganini's violin snapped, and hung down from his instrument. Beads of sweat popped out on his forehead, but he continued playing.

Much to the conductor's surprise, a second string broke, and shortly thereafter, a third. Now there were three limp strings dangling from his violin, but Paganini completed the difficult composition on the one remaining string.

When he finished, the audience jumped to their feet shouting: "Bravo! Bravo!" But Paganini held up his hand to quiet them, and while the audience sank back into their seats, he again picked up his violin.

Holding it high, he nodded to the conductor, and then turned to the crowd and shouted. "Paganini . . . and one string!" After which, he placed the single-stringed Stradivarious beneath his chin and played a magnificent encore.

Likewise, millions of people today are living with broken strings. Most diabetics have only one, a pancreas that refuses to function, but some, like my lady friend, refuse to play on the good strings, preferring instead to complain about their broken string while others, like the blind man in Iowa, make the most of their broken string, continuing on with their lives like nothing ever happened.

If we listen carefully, the soft music generating from that life is absolutely beautiful.

In March, Willy and I attended another three-day School Board Convention in Houston, Texas.

These conventions offer excellent instruction for board members. However, my husband is so aware of the heavy burden placed on taxpayers today that he would not turn a bill in for any of his convention expenses.

His six-year term would expire that fall. He felt he'd served long enough and would not run again for re-election. I was relieved, because it was now consuming so much of his time.

That spring, for the first time in many years, we did not plant cabbage. The closing of the Albro Packing Company mandated that. We were not interested in encroaching upon the New York grower's market, so the closing of that plant was not only a severe blow to our small town, but to area farmers as well.

To fill the gap, we increased our strawberry cultivation to 12 acres. Strawberries are a unique crop, but the blossoms and buds are so tender, that a spring freeze in our part of the country can easily devastate them. In order to protect this crop we installed an irrigation system in our fields.

Most strawberry lovers don't realize that while they are snug in their beds on frosty spring mornings, the strawberry grower has been up most of the night protecting his crop. However, protecting this crop is quite a different matter. Usually, common sense would tell you to just listen to the weather forecast. If the evening temperature was going to drop, then, crank up your irrigation system and let it run until the frost is gone.

Some of you have tasted strawberries where the farmer has done just that, and the first comment you make is, "They don't taste right!" You are absolutely correct. Heavy saturations of water during a strawberry's formation destroys its taste. That's why, large, luscious looking strawberries can taste terrible after a particularly frosty spring.

In order to prevent this, most strawberry farmers talk their wives into checking the temperature for them during those cold evenings. Of course, I was no exception!

Many nights I would begin at midnight, checking the temperature every hour on the hour until the thermometer read 34 degrees. The thermometer wasn't fastened to a window sill, where all I had to do was shine a flashlight on it. No, the thermometer had to be close to the ground, away from buildings to get a correct reading. If I was ever in doubt, we had a spot in our backyard similar to the strawberry patch, where all I had to do was run my fingers over the grass to see if ice had started to form.

When that happened, I immediately called my husband who drove the tractor to the strawberry patch. The largest field was a mile from our house. I followed with the pickup truck.

After hooking the tractor to the irrigation system, we sometimes discovered that the temperature wasn't quite at the freezing point. So, we patiently waited, until frost started to form on the leaves. When that happened, Willy would have to pump the irrigation system by hand until it was primed. Then, as water flowed through the system we carefully checked each sprinkler making sure they turned properly. The heads tend to clog easily, and if they did, we would take a fine piece of wire and unclog the hole, while trying to dodge water from the sprinklers that were turning properly.

It was really a great experience at one, two or three o'clock on those cold, frosty mornings. But our work was well rewarded when the berries set and huge green strawberries started to form.

The following spring we purchased a motor home, which for me eliminated travel frustrations concerning proper refrigeration of my insulin. However, manufacturers now claim insulin need not be refrigerated. Here again, it's always wise to check with your doctor before making a final decision.

That year we drove to Canada on our first fishing trip. After reaching our destination, a fishing camp in the Kipawa region of South Western Quebec, we rented a boat, and spent a frustrating two days fishing. We soon found out that the fishing had been disappointing there most of the summer. The owner of the camp also owned a bush camp, inaccessible by road. He decided to fly out to the camp. We felt very flattered when he invited us to accompany him.

The following day we climbed into a small Beaver airplane equipped with pontoons. After gaining altitude, we thrilled at the lovely forest-covered terrain dotted with numerous lakes. The pilot spotted a big bull moose standing in the wild. Wow! What a fantastic sight.

We landed on the lake and carried our supplies into one of the cabins. What a beautiful setting, seemingly miles away from any civilization. Willy and John explored the area while I unpacked our belongings.

Then, I noticed something else was occupying our cabin; mice! A slow shiver ran down my spine. I decided I'd sleep outside that night, but when

John came running in, telling about the bear manure they discovered around the cabin, I changed my mind.

While the boys were helping Bob, the owner, I rolled up my sleeves, and started to clean the cabin hoping it would chase the scurrying, little creatures outside with the bear. Ah, the joys of nature!

When I finished cleaning, I stepped outside and splashed my feet in the crystal clear lake, marveling again at the flawless beauty of this area.

After a quick supper, Bob navigated us to a favorite fishing spot where Willy caught several walleye. It was late when we got back to camp. I jumped into my sleeping bag hoping the mice wouldn't find me.

It's a good thing my sugar was in good control, because the bathroom was parked outside the cabin in a building they called an out-house. And you'd never catch me using that thing in the middle of the night.

We spent four days fishing in that beautiful area. On our final day Willy and I got up at dawn and hiked a mile up an old logging trail to Little Trout Lake where we found a boat and motor just where Bob said it would be. After shoving off we again marveled at the beautiful scenery while we fished.

Bob intended to ride up the trail on his dirt bike to get the motor after we finished fishing. So to save him the trouble, Willy handed me the fishing poles, along with the fish we'd caught, and started down the trail carrying the motor.

He went so fast I had a hard time keeping up with him, but I hurried along, wondering just what I'd do if one of those big black bears came after my fish? Well, of course, I'd give him the fish, no question about that. But I was glad my worries were unfounded. After a quick breakfast, we watched the airplane land on the water and glide to the dock where we were waiting.

We left Canada that day quite satisfied with our 85-quart cooler filled to the brim with fish.

My year with Dr. Nesbitt was now over, and I was again seeing Dr. Kirkpatrick. After an afternoon appointment, I was waiting while his secretary made my next appointment, and I could see she was having a difficult time working me in.

"If it will help you out, I wouldn't mind going back to Dr. Nesbitt," I offered.

"That would be great," was her reply. So my new friend, Dr. John Nesbitt, was now stuck with me.

Our equipment sheds were bursting at the seams, and to eliminate this, we constructed a large machinery storage building directly behind our barn.

In early October the corn harvest began. It almost seemed like child's play without a cabbage crop to contend with at the same time. That same year, a Conneaut School Board member resigned due to poor health, and the current board members persuaded my husband to come back and fill his existing term.

Each year since the discovery of my diabetes, I've faithfully made a practice of having my eyes examined by an ophthalmologist. In the fall of 1979 I made an appointment with a new eye doctor. There was nothing wrong with my previous ophthalmologist, but ever since this new doctor set up his practice I'd heard excellent reports about him, so I decided to have him examine my eyes.

It was late November when I finally sat in the physician's office filling out the required information sheet for new patients. In the proper block I checked the word diabetic, and in the space provided wrote 32 years.

Soon the doctor's assistant appeared, and gave me the usual sight test to see if I needed a change in my reading glasses. No change was needed. Then, he started a series of drops so the doctor could check my eyes for any signs of diabetic retinopathy.

While waiting for the drops to take effect, I thought how fortunate I'd been all these years to still have such excellent eyesight.

After a short time the new doctor appeared holding my information sheet in his hand. He questioned me emphatically on my long term diabetes, after which, he sat down on his stool, rolled it towards me, and slowly began examining my right eye, then my left eye, and back to my right eye again. Finally, after a long detailed examination, he pushed his stool back, removed his glasses, and while chewing on them said, "You should be blind."

"I want you to go immediately to the Ear & Eye Hospital in Pittsburgh to see a Dr. Gilbert Grand. I'll have my nurse make the appointment for you."

I could scarcely believe what I was hearing. And my mind cried, "No, it can't be true!" However, when I got to the front desk, his nurse was dialing the telephone. Finally, I regained my composure, telling her, "I could not possibly go to Pittsburgh until my husband finished shelling corn."

She put the telephone down, and hurried to talk with the doctor. When she returned, she instructed me to call her just as soon as I was free as my appointment had to be made through that doctor.

When I reached the pickup truck, my fingers were shaking so badly I could barely get the key into the ignition.

"Why did I tell the nurse I couldn't go to Pittsburgh until the corn was harvested?" Willy would be furious with me. "Well, I certainly won't be any blinder a few weeks from now then I am today," I mused. I started my slow, painful drive home while my mind tried desperately to sort this all out. It had just been a year since my last eye exam, and I wondered why the doctor had not given me some kind of a warning then.

Oh, of all the complications this was the one I feared the most. When I pulled into our driveway tears were spilling down my cheeks.

Willy was unloading corn and he walked over to greet me. After seeing my tears, he listened patiently as I told him what happened.

"Why don't you call the nurse tomorrow and have her make the appointment," He suggested, when I finished my woeful tale.

"No, let's finish the corn," I pleaded. Then, he realized just how frightened I was.

It took two weeks before the corn harvest was completed and I'd like to tell you how strong I was during that time. However, I can't. They were in fact the worst two weeks I've ever spent. My husband will also tell you that those weeks were the lowest he'd ever seen me.

All my life I'd lived in dread of diabetic complications, that's why I worked so hard keeping my sugar in good control. Now, it had all been in vain. The enemy I faced is known as DEFEAT!

Moreover, I have always viewed diabetic complications in much the same realm as a thief supposedly threatening me. Of course, I don't know about you, but if I ever saw fingers gripping the window sill in an attempt to enter my house, I'd slam the window down on those fingers. And that's what I'd always tried to do in regards to my diabetes. Let me explain:

When our diabetes is discovered, the fingers of complications are already on our window sill just waiting a chance to enter. They never with-draw, but constantly try to edge closer. That's why it is so important for us to fight this thief with good control. For most diabetic complications occur in people with poor control.

That's the bad news. But the good news is: even when a complication gets in, returning to good control can often minimize its effect.

Early, on December 18, the day of our son's 16th birthday, my husband and I started towards Pittsburgh for my morning appointment with Dr. Grand. While Willy drove, I stared out the window not really seeing anything. All these years I'd taken my eyesight quite for granted, and now that I was losing it, how precious it had become.

We arrived at the Pittsburgh Ear & Eye Hospital with time to spare, and sat in a downstairs waiting room watching children being admitted.

Finally, a nurse appeared and guided us to Dr. Grand's offices where my eyes were examined by an assistant after which, I was escorted upstairs for numerous x-rays, then downstairs again for drops and another examination.

When Dr. Grand finally examined my eyes, his manner was explicitly kind, and I realized that this doctor was touched with blindness everyday.

After my final exam, Dr. Grand checked my x-rays while Willy and I sat in the waiting room next to a woman who had a cancer of the eye. She never said a word, but my heart went out to her and the heavy burden she bore.

Soon, a nurse appeared, and escorted my husband and me into Dr. Grand's office. Willy sat to his left while I sat directly in front of him, bracing myself for the verdict.

When he started to speak, a kind smile flashed across his face, and I thought, "Oh, please don't smile, just tell me." But my thoughts were interrupted when he said, "Mary, I want to congratulate you. I don't know what method you've used to control your diabetes all these years, but however you've done it, you've done it well."

My husband and I exchanged puzzled glances while he went on to explain about diabetic retinopathy.

"It does not occur overnight, there is a process leading up to it with definite stages." (That's why, a yearly examination by a doctor of ophthalmology is extremely important to diabetics). "All I can tell from examining your eyes, is that you are a diabetic. Nothing more!"

Wow! Did you ever really see anyone dance on a ceiling? Well, it definitely happens, because after hearing that, I was literally dancing on the doctor's ceiling.

"But why did the eye doctor send her here?" My husband questioned. "We thought she was going blind!"

Again, Dr. Grand smiled, as he said; "It's not very often we see long term diabetics without some eye damage. I'm quite sure your doctor thought he had missed something, and undoubtedly wanted another opinion."

Then, I questioned Dr. Grand about the cataract in my right eye. He informed me there was also one beginning in my left eye, but according to him, it was no big deal. We'd worry about the cataracts when the time was right.

Dr. Grand mentioned that he would send a detailed report to Dr. Nesbitt, and I chuckled, wondering what my doctor's reaction would be when he read that report. In fact, I could hear him saying; "How did you ever get to the Ear & Eye Hospital in Pittsburgh?" And I'd have a good time telling him.

Willy and I stopped at a favorite Meadville restaurant for a celebration lunch, and we joyfully observed John's birthday with some of his friends that evening.

Nevertheless, while I experienced a joyful release from yet another hardship, it was painfully evident that I had not sought the Lord's council, but had in fact shut him out. Oh, I went through the motions all right, but my defeatist attitude had created a real barrier.

If only, after hearing the eye doctor's comment, I would have committed that worry to God.

However, I didn't do that. Instead, I picked that heavy burden up, choosing to carry it, and all I carried was heavy, excess baggage. Nothing more!

God never forces himself upon us. As Isaiah wrote.

> Therefore the Lord longs to be
> gracious to you. And therefore he
> waits on high to have compassion
> on you. For the Lord is a God of
> Justice; How blessed are all those
> who long for him.
>
> Isaiah 30:18.

How wonderful that God allows us to profit from our mistakes. Likewise, you can be sure, whatever I might be called upon to face in the future, I definitely will not face it alone.

Shortly after my first appointment with Dr. Kirkpatrick, my husband also began seeing him for yearly physicals. One spring afternoon following his checkup, he told me about a new machine Dr's Kirkpatrick and Nesbitt were using to check blood sugars with.

"They just prick your finger; nothing to it," my husband exclaimed! Little did I realize, what an important roll that new machine would someday play in my life.

CHAPTER 14

The Miracle Machine

In February of 1982, Willy and I attended another strawberry grower's conference in Madison, Wisconsin. My husband pampered my love for trains by arranging our trip on Amtrak from Erie to Chicago, whereupon, reaching Chicago we rented a car for our drive to Wisconsin.

When the meetings ended, we drove back to Chicago and spent a day in that city. I'm sure you realize by now that we both love to travel. On this trip I was fascinated with our visit to the Chicago Board of Trade.

What an active lifestyle those brokers have. When I watched all the confusion down below us, I wondered if there might be an insulin-dependent diabetic engaged in that ferocious occupation. If there had been, I would have really enjoyed talking with him or her, to learn how they have adapted their control to that exciting life.

Incidentally, I am not convinced that diabetics need to shun certain lifestyles or occupations because of their "problem." On the contrary, I always encourage them to adjust their control to whatever profession they choose.

In June, our John graduated from high school receiving the Agricultural Award. Now intent on becoming a full-fledged dairy farmer, he rented our barn for his then 10 head of Registered Holsteins, along with 100 acres of farm land from Shadeland, located within a mile of our farm.

Grain prices were now staggering, and farmers everywhere were tightening their belts. It was disheartening watching our markets slip away. Today's politicians have become too much involved in farming. They have promoted too many 'dollar' give away programs for non-production when they should have been making an effort to help secure stable markets around the world for United States farmers.

Many years ago, when the Federal Government started waving their green flags of price supports and programs, it looked wonderful. We, along with many other farmers, signed up to receive money to help pay for some of the drain tile we installed in our wet fields. However, our feelings towards this money soon changed. We realized we could no longer participate in these programs with a good conscience. So we declined them. We were engaged in farming because we loved the land, not because we wanted to be paid for unplanted fields.

Consequently, what started out as a small amount of help for farmers has now grown into monstrous controls by a near bankrupt government. And those of us who have chosen to remain free are now bucking these controls.

Many people view the government as a smiling sugar daddy, who only has to reach into his over-flowing pocket to grant their wishes. In reality, the government is the hard working American taxpayer, with whom I can easily identify.

Today, many farm consultants, along with newspapers and magazines, have developed a new terminology, advising their clients to farm the government. Hearing that phrase hurts me, because in reality, every time someone takes from the federal government they are farming you, me, and themselves.

The real danger in all of this is that someday the politicians promoting this handout are going to scratch their heads, realizing there isn't any more left to give.

A long time ago we heard the phrase: "There's no free lunch." Today, many American farmers are now realizing the true meaning of that phrase.

The real heartbreak of it all is that the free country you and I were blessed to live in will not be passed on to our children. For when officials give, they must also take, and when the well finally runs dry, very few will be able to pay back what they've taken from the government.

At that point our elected representatives will begin taking whatever people have including farms, businesses, etc. to satisfy that debt. Then, of course, the tables will be turned, and our government will farm the people in what was once the greatest free enterprising country in the world.

In 1983 Dr. John Nesbitt talked to me about a Blood Glucose Monitoring Machine. "I'd really like you to try one," He suggested. And I never dreamed what that one machine would eventually do for my control.

If you are not familiar with a Blood Glucose Monitoring Machine, it is a machine that can automatically determine a person's blood glucose level. Let me explain how it works:

After washing and thoroughly drying your hands, you press the machine's On/Off button, then, prick the side of your finger to obtain a large drop of blood. At that point, you press the time button on the machine and immediately apply the drop of blood to the proper test strip.

In approximately 40 seconds you will need to blot the test strip in accordance with the machine's instructions, most will offer warning beeps at the proper blotting time. Raise the test strip hatch, and place the test strip into the hatch closing it securely. After the display meter reaches "00" the meter will automatically determine your correct blood glucose level, and the result will appear in the display. The entire process takes only 60 seconds.

Most machines are small enough to fit into a womans' purse, and these machines are now available without a prescription at most pharmacies.

At that time there were many different machines on the market.

My husband and I carefully researched them with the help of our local Diabetes Associations to find the right machine for me.

We first attended a meeting at City Hospital in Meadville, Pennsylvania where a nurse presented a program on the machines. Afterwards, diabetics were welcome to have their blood glucose level tested by the nurse.

That night I was amazed at the significantly high blood glucose levels some diabetics were carrying. My heart went out to a lovely teenage girl, who was absolutely crushed when her blood glucose level read 300, and another woman, probably in her mid-forties whose blood glucose level was 400.

The woman sat across from Willy and me and told us she was swimming at the YWCA to try and correct the problem. However, she was also at odds with her doctor because of those high blood glucose levels. I soon discovered that this is a rather common problem among some diabetics.

Oh, how I had to restrain myself, because I desperately wanted to slip my arm around the woman, and explain the danger of carrying a 400 blood sugar in her system for any length of time. I also wanted to remind her that exercise would not bring down a 400 blood sugar. In fact, it probably only aggravated it. In my opinion, she desperately needed to take the required amount of Regular Insulin to help bring it down to an acceptable level.

We've talked considerably about low blood sugars. But what do we do about those high blood sugars?

Of course, we all wish they would never occur because they are such a serious problem. In this case wishing does not make it so. As much as we hate them, they do occur. However, minimizing their occurrences should be of extreme importance to us.

When I was young, Dr. Stoney had a strict rule about 4-plus urine sugars. I'm sure you old timers remember them. They were a vivid orange color. His rule was quite simple. He just would not tolerate them!

Now there can be many reasons besides overeating which cause a high blood glucose level. A head cold or any minor illness like a virus or the flu. Also, an infection or an incorrect insulin calculation, even stress can sometimes be the culprit.

Nevertheless, when high blood sugars occur, what do we do about them? Dr. Stoney's rule some 40 years ago was to always treat a 4-plus urine sugar with 10 units of Regular Insulin. Of course, after doing that, I had to stay home, continually testing until my urine sugar reached negative. But many times that 10 units was way too much insulin, and I then had to recorrect it with additional food.

However, when I purchased a Blood Glucose Monitoring Machine, the uncertain knowledge that I'd used for so many years to treat an occasional high blood sugar changed, to a very reliable, dependable method. I was so impressed with this machine, and what it did for my control that I named mine The Miracle Machine.

Let's face it, we all hope we'll never need to correct a high blood sugar, but if we ever do the Miracle Machine can help us do it correctly.

Remember, we are all different, and the calculation I use might not be right for you, but working with your doctor, along with careful testing on a Blood Glucose Monitoring Machine will allow you to determine a correct calculation for yourself.

Let me explain mine: If I checked my

blood glucose level at eight o'clock in the evening, and happened to find it running at 240, I would immediately take 4 units of Regular Insulin, allowing one unit of insulin for every 25 points of blood sugar above 140, which, in a very short time (2–4 hours) would bring my blood glucose level down to approximately 140. Now, I don't want it any lower because I have a long-acting insulin working overnight in my body, and I do not want to throw myself into an insulin reaction. As a result, between six thirty and seven o'clock the following morning, my blood glucose level will usually read between 70 and 80.

Again, I must caution you never to attempt a correction without your doctor's knowledge until you've become thoroughly experienced in the proper correction technique for yourself.

Today, with the proper use of a Miracle Machine, you and I can experience near perfect control. I just can't say enough for this machine. It was undoubtedly the missing link in the chain of good diabetic control. I only wish Dr. George Stoney could have lived to see that chain made perfect.

Once in a while a diabetic will tell me that they just can't get their blood sugar under control. Brittle is the term used when a diabetic suffers from wide swings in blood glucose levels. However, these cases are extremely rare. Sometimes we need to try just a little harder to get those blood sugars under control.

I still experience days when, for no apparent reason, my blood sugar tends to run low, and occasionally, a day when I have to fight a high blood sugar. If you experience the same tendencies, don't let it beat you, but work patiently until you develop the perseverance it takes to stabilize those days.

A few years ago I received a letter from Dr. Gilbert Grand conveying a sad message. He was accepting a position at Barrer Hospital in St. Louis, Missouri, and would be leaving Pittsburgh to fill that position.

After receiving that message I hesitantly started back to my previous ophthalmologist. However, I was not satisfied, especially, after one exam when he took numerous x-rays of my right eye to check for signs of retinopathy because the cataract was now blocking his ability to see properly.

It was now blocking my vision even more than I wanted to admit. It was difficult for me to read or do any of my bookwork without the aid of a magnifying glass.

Driving had also become difficult, as my son can tell you. One afternoon I picked him up at one of our fields east of town, and while driving home, almost hit a mauve colored vehicle coming towards us. I just did not see it! If John had not hollered in time, it might have been disastrous.

It was then a dear friend highly recommended a Dr. Barry Stamm in Erie, Pennsylvania. And I immediately made an appointment with Dr. Stamm.

In February of 1984 Dr. Stamm examined my eyes. He was every bit as kind as Dr. Grand, realizing what a frightening experience it was for me to commit the care of my precious eyesight to a perfect stranger.

However, after a few minutes with Dr.

Stamm, I realized, like so many others, that I could trust him. Surgery for the cataract in my right eye was scheduled at 11:30 A.M. on March 13, at Hamot Hospital in Erie.

Dr. Stamm instructed me to take my insulin and eat a light breakfast before going to the hospital. After arriving at Hamot, I went through a series of pre-admission tests, including a vein-type blood test. While the technician sought to find a good vein, my heart rejoiced at the thought of my Miracle Machine which ended that once terrible ordeal of vein type blood tests for me.

After being admitted, my husband sat with me trying to relax my concern over the injection which would numb my eye for the surgery. (Yes, I'm still a terrible coward). Moreover, I'd frightened myself by listening to people tell how terrible this injection is. As usual, my fears were unfounded. It was no different than the occasional novacaine I receive at my dentist's office.

During surgery, Dr. Stamm removed the affected lens, and replaced it with a plastic lens, because, when the lens is removed from an eye, it makes the eye markedly farsighted. The plastic lens would hopefully correct this condition.

He released me from the hospital the following morning. I continued following the instructions given me. I saw Dr. Stamm at regular intervals after that and my eye healed beautifully.

Dr. Stamm also sent a detailed report to Dr. Nesbitt as it's always important that the doctors caring for us maintain good communication.

On November 27, of that same year, the cataract in my left eye was removed on an out-patient basis, allowing me once again to enjoy the perfect vision I'd lost to cataracts.

Once a year Dr. Stamm carefully examines my eyes, paying special attention to any signs of retinopathy that might occur in this long term diabetic. At my last appointment he was extremely pleased. Don't disdain good control. Remember, it pays.

Usually, there will be a waiting period before seeing any good doctor for the first time unless, of course, you are suffering a dire emergency. However, today, if you were to call any of the Dr. Kirkpatricks, Dr. Nesbitts, or Dr. Stamms the world over, you will be required to wait until their schedule can accommodate you. Please take my advice, your wait will be well worth it.

Today, with the careful use of a Miracle Machine, my insulin has been reduced a full 10 units. The only trouble I've experienced from a really low blood sugar happened quite unexpectantly one evening.

On a sunny April morning in 1985, I cleaned my freezer, and had 18 quarts of frozen, sugarless strawberries to use before our new crop arrived. I rolled up my sleeves and began making strawberry jelly, stirring one large batch after the other, carefully sealing each jar with paraffin. This was the first time I had ever made cooked strawberry jelly because freezer jam is much easier.

It was a long day, but the 46 jars of jelly looked beautiful sitting on my kitchen counter. While I was drying the last large pan, Willy stuck his head in the kitchen door, asking me if I wanted to go for a ride with him to Shadeland.

Oh, that sounded wonderful! So I grabbed

my sweater, dashed out the door and climbed into our pickup truck.

John was chisel plowing in a back field, a mile from the main road. His dad wanted to see how soon he would finish plowing that field.

It was just about dark when we entered the long driveway, running from one field to the other. In the middle of that drive was a small swamp, still swelled from the early spring rains. There, our four-wheel drive pickup bottomed out and simply would not move.

John had a tractor only a few feet away, but no chain with which to pull out the truck. Willy decided to walk home. I was bound and determined to walk with him. I searched the glove compartment of the pickup where I usually keep something sweet for emergencies. Then, I recalled cleaning out the glove compartment and had not yet restocked it.

"Oh, I can make it," I pleaded. "A walk will really do me good after that long day in the kitchen." However, Willy was not convinced. He urged me to walk back and watch John plow while he was gone, but I insisted on walking home with him.

"Okay," he finally agreed, "let's try it." Yes, his reasoning was correct. He knows how carefully I control my blood sugar and he also knows what exercise can do without extra food to counteract it.

Nevertheless, we started through the field, and down the old Penn Central railroad bed rather enjoying our unexpected walk. However, after a mile-and-a-half I knew I was in trouble. And we still had a half mile to go. We were now up on the dirt road, but there is only one house on that road, and it was pitch-dark.

"Just a half mile to go," I kept telling myself, while Willy urged me to climb up on his back to conserve whatever energy I had left, but I wouldn't hear of it! Oh, how stubborn I am!

"I can make it, I can make it," I kept telling him, trying to convince myself as well. But he knew better.

Finally, I was staggering so badly Willy knelt down, and hoisted me across his back where he could easily carry me. Oh, if only I had cooperated earlier, because I soon began flopping, and flailing, making it utterly impossible for him to walk with me.

He considered placing me beside a large oak tree while he went for something sweet. But he quickly changed his mind fearful I might crawl away in my confused condition and he would not be able to find me.

At that point, he held my arms together, literally dragging me down the road and across the Beaver Center blacktop, finally placing me near a telephone pole in one of the fields we'd recently planted to strawberries, only a few hundred feet from our house.

He ran for the tractor which was parked at the irrigation system in that field, and drove to where I was sitting. After hoisting me up, he quickly drove home where he grabbed a piece of bread, and immediately covered it with strawberry jelly. Then, he held me upright on the tractor while I slowly munched on the soft bread and jelly.

After all these years he knows I can no longer stand orange juice with sugar. Oh, how I love that man!

In just a few minutes the jelly took effect.

Afterwards, as Willy recounted our walk, I shuddered, grateful I had not started out alone. But maybe, just maybe, we all need a close call once in a while to remind ourselves that we must constantly be on guard. However, that kind of experience should only happen once every 40 years.

Thinking back, if only I had grabbed my purse or jammed something into my pocket that evening, my husband and I could have enjoyed a lovely romantic walk. But I was caught short! No doubt about it.

When people leave home they usually presume that they will return without incident. That evening I learned a never-to-be forgotten lesson in presumption. In fact, I've stricken the word from my diabetic vocabulary.

The American Express Card people have a snappy little advertisement telling us: "Don't leave home without it." I now appropriate their advertisement every time I head for the door, reminding myself of the unusual predicaments diabetics can encounter. You can be sure I'll never leave home without it, again: the "it," of course, being something with which to counteract an insulin reaction.

One evening at a local Diabetes Association meeting, Willy and I watched a young mother check her son's blood glucose level.

The boy was six years old, and had been diagnosed with diabetes since the age of three. His glucose level was extremely high, and she chatted about sending him to a diabetic camp that summer so he could get in good control.

Diabetic camps are helpful and encouraging, however, good control must be practiced daily. You don't just "get" in good control. It is a constant effort. His mother continued chatting about this and that, seemingly unaware that she held the real key to this child's control.

Oh, she was going through the motions all right. But something was missing. With a blood sugar as high as that child was carrying, he definitely needed more insulin.

There is a regimentation with which diabetics must live, but many choose to ignore the regimentation. If that's your choice, fine. But don't go through some of the motions while ignoring the real key to success in this walk, which is simply doing the correct thing to treat your blood glucose level.

Of course, we all know that for a low blood glucose level, food is required. Remember, a moderate blood glucose level can be brought down safely with exercise and careful eating. However, a high blood glucose level of 300 or more always demands insulin.

We all make mistakes, but with the careful use of our Blood Glucose Monitoring Machine we can usually rectify those mistakes. Nevertheless, one young man was not so fortunate, and it was the announcement of his tragic death that finally persuaded me to begin this book.

He was only 19, and beginning his freshman year at an Erie college. He lived in Pittsburgh, and during his first week in Erie, drowned while swimming in Lake Erie. The newscaster reported that he was a diabetic and an insulin reaction was highly suspected as the cause of his death.

My heart cried for him for I could associate my young energies of years past along with my love for swimming with him. I tried to force back the

207

tears, when I pictured the trauma he must have suffered after his strength from an insulin reaction failed, and he could not make it back to shore.

We all get up against it at times! I could have easily understood this happening in prior years. But today . . . no, not with Blood Glucose Monitoring Machines so easily available to us. However, they won't do us any good if we don't use them.

Most exercise events are preplanned, and you and I have the option of reducing our insulin, or eating to bring our blood glucose level up to an acceptable level. Never go in swimming with a normal blood glucose, for swimming is not a sport you can mess around with or treat safely when finished. Water can be dangerous!

If you've already taken your insulin injection, eat something to get your blood glucose level up to an acceptable level. Then, if you don't swim enough to bring it down, correct it with another exercise or less food later.

We can live normal healthy lives, but it takes a few extra precautions on our part. The final rule, of course, is never swim alone.

With a Blood Glucose Monitoring Machine we actually hold in our hands the tool for near perfect control. It is because of this machine that you can enjoy a wonderful new hope which was not available to me. If I made it 40 years, struggling 36 of those years without a machine, then those of you who will employ your machine correctly should easily double my years.

That's right! With good control diabetics today can now look forward to a normal life expectancy. Something else will probably get you long before the diabetes does.

Today, some 40 years after the discovery of my diabetes, I am still a very healthy woman. In October my husband and I celebrated 25 years of a wonderful marriage.

Our John is a tall, strong young man, who begins each day at 4:30 A.M., often going non-stop until nine or ten o'clock in the evening. He now has over 100 head of Registered Holsteins and continues to pursue his dream in this area of agriculture.

If you are a new diabetic, please don't be frightened by that diagnosis. Instead, latch on to a control program that works well for you, and live with it. Above all, keep the faith. Perhaps a break-through will come in the not too distant future for all diabetics.

On May 30, 1985, the small town of Albion, Pennsylvania, just a 10-minute drive from us, and the tiny town of Atlantic in our county were struck by separate, devastating tornadoes.

Lives were snuffed out and hundreds of people lost every earthly possession they owned. Three weeks later as fire sirens screeched, we watched from our cellar door as the slender funnel shaped cloud headed straight towards our farm. Suddenly, the tornado veered to the left and dissipated within 300 yards of our house!

God never promised any of us an easy walk on this earth, only a safe harbor to those who will place their faith and trust in Him.

> For God so loved the world, that
> he gave his only begotten Son,
> that whosoever believeth in Him
> should not perish, but have
> everlasting life.
>
> John 3:16.

I've willingly shared with you the serious problems experienced during my 40-year walk with diabetes. Two happened during pregnancies, one from carelessness, and the last one simply because I was unprepared. How I hope you will learn from my mistakes.

When I think of our diabetic walk it often reminds me of the high-wire act seen at the circus, because every time I watch high-wire performers, I am fearful they will fall. Likewise, that's the way most spectators view our diabetic life. It looks absolutely terrifying to them. Most people are frightened of it.

Yet, most high-wire performers are not concerned at all for they have learned to balance correctly. Also, there is usually a safety net beneath them.

Now some performers won't use a safety net, and I refuse to watch them because they appear quite foolish to me.

However, today's diabetic can now walk safely on the high-wire by carefully balancing their insulin, exercise, and eating. Most of us have also discovered that it's not bad at all on the wire.

Perhaps it was a problem at first, but as we've adjusted its become much easier. And we are extremely fortunate to have a dependable instrument to guide us, known as the Blood Glucose Monitoring Machine. It not only helps secure our balance, but in addition, it provides a wonderful safety net for us to live within. Consequently, that once difficult, high-wire walk can now be mastered by any diabetic willing to try.

Of course, we'll fall every once in a while, but as soon as we hit the net we need only climb back onto the wire regaining our careful balance.

How wonderful it is to now live in this technically advanced age of diabetes management that gives us new hope for living with a broken string.

The grass withers, the flower
fades, but the word of our God
shall stand forever.

Isaiah 40:8.

Scripture quotations are taken from
the Scofield Reference Bible, and
the New American Standard Bible.
Copyright, 1909, 1917, 1937, 1945
Oxford University Press.
1960, 1962, 1963, 1971
The Lockman Foundation.

My appreciation to Ames Division of Miles Laboratory
for permission to adapt material from DITN Mailbox
Section, Diabetes In The News, Page 46, March/April
1986 issue.